Robust Vitality

Robust Vitality

An Exploration into the Vibrancy of Being

by Julian James DeVoe

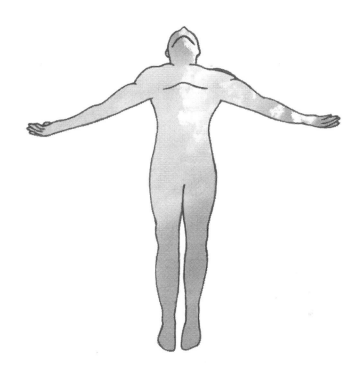

Printed in the United States of America

ISBN-13: 978-1542406239
ISBN-10: 1542406234

Cover and Interior Design: Ghislain Viau
Illustrations: Lisa-Marie Long

Knowledge is power – when you use it constructively.
—David J. Schwartz, Ph. D.

Contents

Acknowledgements

Even though I am the author of this text, it is not all original, nor has it come about solely by my own efforts — the proper acknowledgments must be given.

My father, for helping to deliver my message. Lisa-Marie Long, who helped make it come alive with her artwork. Katy Cox, for her direct contributions and friendship. To those that have helped on my healing journey: Dr. Matt Goltl, Dr. Helen Law and Paul Kelly who continually aid my healing journey; Dr. Nagi Iskander and Karen Whiffen, my Cranio Sacral mentors; Avianna Castro, psychic advisor; Grace Van Berkum, colleague and friend; Michael Sage, who stimulated my physical, mental and spiritual pursuits. To the many wise and inspiring teachers: Shivanter Singh, who has been a supportive teacher and friend. Mukti, Michael Buck, Vedic Thai Massage artist who has shared with me the power of touch. Don Stapleton, Ph.D and Amba who brought to my attention the gift of listening and Self-Awakening Yoga Therapeutics. Shannon Garvey, my first yoga teacher; Hojoung and Andrew Appello, who re-energized my yoga pursuits; and Naime Jezzeny and Sue Elkind, my current teachers. My friends — you know who you are. My immediate family: Sylvia and James (Mom and Dad), Kryssa, Chris, Liliana and Matteo for their unconditional love and support. My extended family.

Robust Vitality

And to all the other countless teachers and students who have contributed to my growth and development.

This work is dedicated to them — without them, none of this would be possible. With grace and gratitude, these teachings are offered.

"healthy." I wasn't looking for anything else. I was tired of feeling "out of whack." (Then I pondered, what does "in whack," feel like? Either way, I was whacked.) Could I go a day without cramps or indigestion? The inquiry of getting "to normal" opened up a door of uncertainty and the unknown.

The upset stomachs angered me so much that I forced myself to change. This was the hardest part of the whole process — change. My anger was the catalyst for this change and a useful one at that. It was time to take charge of my own wellbeing — and thus the journey began. The inquiry into robust vitality began with my body and then moved into my mind and emotions.

My mother suggested I see a colon specialist, so I did. I was diagnosed with irritable bowel syndrome (IBS) — like I really needed a doctor to tell me that — and was given a bottle of over the counter stomach aid, i.e. the pink stuff. I was also instructed to avoid the foods that caused me pain. So, I guess it was back to apples and crackers.

My mother then insisted that I see a homeopathic doctor, so I did. He asked me a few questions about my diet, but more about my work, family, relationships, aspirations and habits (my habits were that of a social drinker and semi-regular pot smoker). It took his questions for me to make the connection about my food (and lifestyle choices) and how I felt. The homeopath took the overall perspective on health and then prescribed a "remedy" that would help. This was my first interaction with "alternative" methods to healing.

I saw the homeopath a few more times and I slowly began to feel better. He encouraged different eating patterns, avoiding things I loved like pizza, meat and balsamic vinegar. He pushed me to re-evaluate my lifestyle choices, occupation and personal relationships. I started reading about diet and nutrition. I made sure to exercise regularly, and began reading self-improvement books.

I went to see an acupuncturist to help with my allergies. After one visit I saw relief in the symptoms that I was told by allergy specialists were incurable. After several sessions the change was significant and all but permanent. Other *side effects* from this method were improved circulation, increased mental clarity and more overall energy.

The shift had been made and I began pursuing alternative forms of therapy: energy workers, massage therapists, several acupuncturists and spiritual healers. I even traveled to the Amazon rainforest in Peru to work with indigenous shamans. My stomach problems were far less frequent, most of my allergies began to clear up, my IBS was gone, my addictions vanished and I started to experience higher levels of happiness and joy. In the process, my body began to tone as well. I never knew that if I focused on my insides that I could develop the body I always wanted.

After a job change (maybe my former boss was right about him making me sick), more ailments dissipated. I had more energy, was sleeping better and much of my anxiety went away. I then started working with a spiritual teacher and he took my health to a whole new level. He guided me through parasite cleanses, liver flushes, colon cleanses heavy metal detoxification and suggested a daily meditation practice and to clear the clutter out of my house. My energy levels sky-rocketed and my entire view on health changed. Instead of seeing health as merely preventing disease, it became a quest for thriving health, total mental, emotional and spiritual fulfillment — for *Robust Vitality.*

Four years after paying attention to my upset stomach, *Robust Vitality* was born.

It has been such a transformative journey personally and professionally. I can now enjoy most foods, even pizza and dessert, without pain. I can be outside during all seasons and play with my dog without sneezing or itchiness. What has been the most thrilling is witnessing countless people change their lives through the simple techniques that are outlined in this manual. I am excited to share these practices because I have experienced their power.

I am excited to be your advocate on this journey. I offer my unwavering support and hope to inspire you to inspire yourself.

Introduction

The key to growth is the introduction of higher dimensions
of consciousness into our awareness.
—Lao Tzu

What is Robust Vitality?

To enjoy *robust vitality* means to thrive on all levels, to experience your fullest potential and to have a healthy, vibrant human experience daily. Each of us has the potential to live a happy, hearty, disease free life. Our birthright is freedom, action and happiness, all of which must be embrace actively or they can be lost.

The human experience is colorful and mysterious to say the least. We are unique multi-dimensional beings that are cooking in a soup of our past events, present temperament and our future ruminations. We exist in varying times and places to greet the present moment with the fullness and totality of who we are. Though our bodies live in the present our thoughts and emotions often to do not. To experience *robust vitality* it is important to sharpen our awareness on what is life affirming and to explore what needs to be refined. We all have areas of dormant vitality that can be awakened, so let's wake them up!

As we exercise our "awareness muscle," it is useful to remember that just like the body's muscles, awareness must be built through stamina, working toward goals and accepting any soreness along the way. Creating new habits takes practice and patience. Consider *Robust Vitality* as an invitational aid, a supplement and a complement to what you have already experienced. Honor yourself, your body's innate wisdom and all your experiences by considering the viewpoint that everything you need to awaken is stored within.

Despite what you might think, you are as perfect as you are just in this moment — breathe that in. What you have, what you have done, what you look and feel like are just enough. Though you are just "right" as you are in the moment, you can grow, evolve and expand. Congratulations, you are the most amazing you the world has seen yet. You are the embodiment of all your experiences and isn't that great, being perfectly imperfect.

Emotional bliss, mental clarity and physical vibrancy are all aspects of what it means to have *robust vitality*. This manual is a combination of techniques, suggestions and information for achieving ultimate/optimal states of vitality. Derived from a variety of spiritual traditions, secular sources, age-old techniques and scientific research, this *Robust Vitality* will cover key components for maximizing your health, your *robust vitality*.

Where do we begin? How do we approach such a quest? Why? What are our motivations? The story below is a useful metaphor for contextualizing how we begin to exercise our muscle of awareness:

A Cherokee is telling his grandson about a fight that is going on inside him. He said it is between two wolves.

One wolf is 'evil': Anger, envy, sorrow, regret, fearful thinking, greed, arrogance, self-pity, guilt, resentment, inferiority, lies, false pride, superiority and ego.

The other wolf is 'good': Joy, peace, love, hope, serenity, humility, kindness, benevolence, empathy, generosity, truth, compassion and faith.

The grandson thought about it for a minute and then asked his grandfather, "Which wolf wins?"

The Cherokee simply replied, "The one I feed."

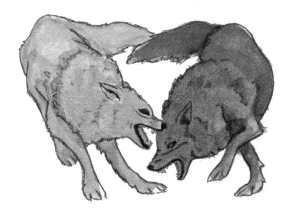

This story points to an inner struggle, in which most of us are engaged. By cultivating vibrant habits (feeding the good wolf), we can increase our self-control and dramatically improve our health. When we fuel our bad habits (the evil wolf), we jeopardize our overall health. By investigating which one we are feeding and why, we can get closer to our authentic self and what it truly needs. By focusing on supercharging our bodies, our good wolf will always be victorious. This is not to say that the evil wolf does not serve a purpose. We can use it as an indicator to teach us what we want to refine or enhance. They will continue to exist in creative tension and are of importance in building our complete self.

In Eckhart Tolle's book, *The New Earth,* he discusses similar concepts found in all major religions. He speaks about two commonalities that they all share:

1. There is a dysfunction that lies within humans that can corrupt itself and others. In the Hindu tradition it is called *maya,* or the veil of illusion. Buddhist traditions call it *dukha* or suffering. Christian teachings discuss the notion of original sin (which when translated from the Greek means to miss the mark — in other words to become misaligned).

2. There is the ability for "radical transformation of consciousness," also known as enlightenment, liberation, awakening or salvation.

His description is similar to the metaphor used by the Native American elder. Recognizing both aspects of ourselves, the question remains: what path do we choose? What attributes do we want to cultivate? How do we nurture them?

However described, there are two pathways where our health and consciousness can lead: toward liberation (the good wolf) or into despair (the evil wolf). By cluing into our inner wisdom we can use our intellect to guide our actions, our heart to motivate and our guts to align us with truth. Shedding 'untruth,' goal setting, community, self-study and dedication will help propel us on this exploration.

Why would you want *robust vitality* and is it even possible? Another way of saying this is: what are your intentions, goals and fears? What do you want and how badly do you want it? What are you willing to do to get it? How open are you to change?

Change is not necessarily easy, but it surely is worth it. It's not easy because our brains have created neural networks for us to do the things that we do with ease. Essentially, the more we do something, the stronger the network, i.e. the faster and easier it is for us, just like traveling along a multi-lane highway. When we change our habits and patterns, we are create new, less traveled pathways, like a dirt road. Over time, we can turn unpaved roads into super highways and deconstruct highways of bad habit altogether. Changing our neural pathways is what scientists call neuroplasticity — it's great news for those of us 'old dogs' wanting to learn new tricks. We just need a little bit of willpower to start.

Motivating ourselves to change can come from many sources. If it comes from a place of fear, that is ok. It is a good place to start, but once your fears (symptoms, anxieties, stresses, stomach aches, weight loss, etc.) are resolved, what then will be your motivator? Since good and bad co-exist in each of us some of these fears will return, some will fester, all will need attention.

Healing your body is only one part of the journey, growing into the fullest expression of physical, mental and spiritual health is next. By reconnecting with our wise (and sacred) core and remembering our life force potential (divine source), it is possible to enjoy and sustain unabiding *robust vitality*.

I am honored and privileged to offer this material to you.

Chapter 1

Starting Off

Nature is infinitely creative.
It is always producing the possibility of new beginnings.
—Marianne Williamson

We begin our pursuit by determining exactly where we *are*. This section is designed to give us perspective on figuring out where to start and what direction to take. It is an overview of concepts that will help us throughout the exploration of *robust vitality*. We will touch on components that will be discussed more deeply in later sections.

The Power of Process

Throughout this reading and experimentation things in your life may shift and change. Not all of it will come with ease or fluidity. Knowing that there may be challenges and difficulties is part of the *process* — the process of transformation. To help us navigate through these experiences is a guide created by Don Stapleton, Ph.D. called the *Cycle of Awareness*. Stapleton developed this model as part of the Self Awakening Yoga® coursework curriculum.

CYCLE OF AWARENESS

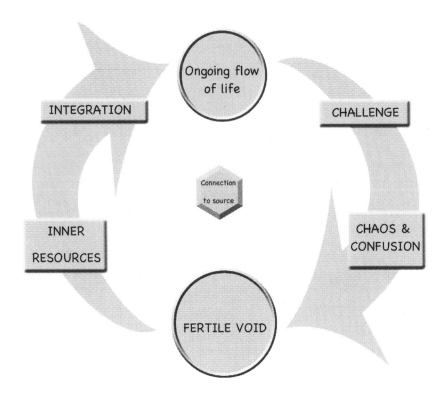

- Normal ongoing flow of life, day-to-day. Being present and witnessing our experience.
- A challenge intersects with our normal flow. This opportunity can cause a shift that may knock us off balance. Our relationship to the challenge is what is significant, not whether it is perceived as a major life event, or something small.
- Finding a way to accept the confusion and chaos will help us embrace the experience. As Stapleton notes, allowing it to be "as messy as it actually is." We don't have to fight or change our experience to bring us back to normal; but rather, witness it and ourselves in it.
- Entering the fertile void is the place of letting go into self-awareness. Allowing ourselves to be with the unknown.
- The place of inner resources is where we see options. We can embrace intuition, be creative and lean on inner knowing.

- Integration occurs when we take in the lessons learned and grow through them. New practices, habits and ideas can lead into a new evolved state of being.
- Evolution into a new state of being is when we fully awaken into a new place of wholeness.

The *Cycle of Awareness* speaks to the power of process and how we can see clearly the stages of change and growth. In my personal experience this process is happening all the time for different things and with varying degrees of intensity. Being able to put my finger on where I am in the process has helped me settle into my experience rather than wish to be somewhere other than where I am.

Vital Nutrients:
What Are You Hungry For?

Shivanter Singh, health coach and graduate of the Institute of Integrative Nutrition (IIN), spoke about the concept of "primary foods." He would start his nutrition discussion with the question: what are primary foods? Common answers are fruits, vegetables, grains and meat/fish/poultry. Many health advocates now consider these edible foods to be a secondary source of nutrition.

So, if edible food is a secondary source of nutrition, than what are *Vital Nutrients?* What then are we actually hungry for; and how are we supposed to feed ourselves? It is less of a question and more of a riddle because the concept of *vital nutrients* expands the definition of food and nutrition to include our mental, emotional and spiritual needs. Things such as relationships, creativity, finances, sex life, career and spiritual practice are all considered sources of nutrition.

I really love this inquiry because it forces us stretch our "awareness muscle" to redefine our concept of food. In homeopathy, doctors take a holistic approach to health that evaluates *vital nutrients*. The Ayurvedic System (the Indian system for health, healing and eating) has a similar concept of evaluating lifestyle behaviors. To limit our definition of health and hunger to only edibles, we miss much of what constitutes health.

Do we really want that macaroni and cheese; or do we want that hug from mom? Are we really craving sweets; or do we want the sweetness of a creatively fulfilled life? Is it the extra cup of coffee, or an energizing conversation that we really desire?

Sometimes when we get inspired and enter "the zone," when we are passionately in love or engrossed in our natural environment, the sensations of hunger are minimal. We are being fueled by *vital nutrients.* Other times, when feeling upset or depressed, we emotionally eat, yet no amount of food can satisfy our needs. The opposite is also true, have you ever been "love sick" after a break-up or a loss of a relative. Hunger was never even felt. What we are craving during these times are *vital nutrients.* A hug, a lively conversation or a work project may be the vitamins and minerals we need. No matter how much we eat, or don't eat, fulfillment comes through other means.

What was different during those times? What made time slip by and hunger absent? It was because we were feeding on *vital nutrients.* In fact, there are some people that can go long periods of time without edibles at all. There are documented cases of people not eating for months on end. One famous example of this is the "starving yogi," a man whom claims to have not consumed food or water for over 70 years.[1] After spending almost 2 weeks in a hospital, under heavy surveillance (and scrutiny) by doctors, scientists and the military, no one could explain how he did it. He had baffled them. This is an extreme example of a primary nutritionist; and it's fascinating to consider the human capacity to thrive without edibles.

Most spiritual practices encourage a process of fasting or abstinence; so that believers can pay tribute to their core needs — dining on *vital nutri-ents.* It not only allows the body to clean itself, but also allows for dining on divinity. For Christians, Lent is such a practice and stories of Jesus fasting in the desert are well known. Jews observe Yom Kippur, a period of fasting for the sake of atonement — as one of my friends says, "at-One-ment." Muslims observe Ramadan every year by fasting during the day.

---

1 http;// Physa.org/news.html

One of the greatest experiences I have had to dine via *vital nutrients* was during a vision quest in the Black Hills of South Dakota. I spent 3 days without food or water, delving into other things that sustain me. Not only did abstinence sustain me, but it also made me thrive — there are things that are greater than physical needs. One of my main and most fulfilling meals was gratitude.

All too often we project mental, emotional and/or spiritual needs on our food choices. When we look around the American society, we see an epidemic of obesity. What *is* really happening? It *is* a lack of *vital nutrients*. Most Americans are hungry and craving nutrition, but not the kind that comes from food. The problem of obesity is largely due to deficiencies in mental, emotional and spiritual nutrition. To be fed by *vital nutrients* like a creative project, prayer, enjoying a book or being passionately involved with a lover is often more satisfying than a meal.

It is worth repeating: what makes you hungry?

The Quality of Life Inventory and Wheel of Vitality exercises are two ways to come in closer contact with what it is that you are actually craving. They are fast and simple exercises that will help you make better food choices from life's menu.

Quality of Life Inventory

The following exercise comes from a beloved teacher, Vedic Thai Yoga massage artist Mukti (Michael Buck). Grace and gratitude to him for passing along this wonderful technology. The *Quality of Life Inventory* process was composed by a think-tank of psychologists who considered the question: what determines quality of life? They came up with a list of essential qualities that determine our state of being. This list has been updated and modified several times since its original incarnation.

Directions

1. Ascribe a number from 1-10 for each of the 13 categories. 1 is the lowest quality rating and 10 indicates the highest quality rating.

2. Add the numbers together and divide the total by 13. The resulting number represents your Quality of Life Inventory calculation.

3. If you desire to improve the quality of your life but do not know where to start, this exercise will help. Pick one or two categories to improve and think creatively about how you want to facilitate the change.

This exercise is a tremendous asset because it provides insight, 'at a glance,' at how we feel about ourselves. Daily, weekly or monthly we can repeat this process and see where and how we are progressing. Having an assessment by someone who is familiar with you, like a close friend, family member or partner can be a valuable part of the practice. Remember it is only a number. (The quotes are inspirational passages about the category; they do not pertain to the actual practice.)

1. Attitude

"Keep your thoughts positive because your thoughts become your words. Keep your words positive because your words become your behavior. Keep your behavior positive because your behavior becomes your habits. Keep your habits positive because your habits become your values. Keep your values positive because your values become your destiny." —Mahatma Gandhi

2. Posture

"A good stance and posture reflect a proper state of mind." —Morihei Ueshiba

3. Structure

"Do you wish to be great? Then begin by being. Do you desire to construct a vast and lofty fabric? Think first about the foundations of humility. The higher your structure is to be, the deeper must be its foundation." —Saint Augustine

4. Contribution

"We make a living by what we get. We make a life by what we give." —Winston Churchill

5. Exercise

"A bear, however hard he tries, grows tubby without exercise." —A.A. Milne

6. Rest/Relaxation

"It's a good idea always to do something relaxing prior to making an important decision in your life." —Paulo Coelho

7. Diet/Nutrition

"Eat food. Not too much. Mostly plants." —Michael Pollan

8. Fun

"I know it is wet and the sun is not sunny, but we can have lots of good fun that is funny." —Dr. Seuss

9. Sex

"Sex is the most fun you can have without laughing." —Woody Allen

10. Money

"A Penny Saved is a Penny Earned" —Benjamin Franklin

11. Dharma/Purpose

"He who has a why to live for can bear almost any how." —Friedrich Nietzsche

12. Relationships

"The meeting of two personalities is like the contact of two chemical substances: if there is any reaction, both are transformed." —C.G. Jung

13. Spirituality

"Make your own Bible. Select and collect all the words and sentences that in all your readings have been to you like the blast of a trumpet." —Ralph Waldo Emerson

The Wheel of Vitality

This exercise will help you to discover which primary foods you are missing the most. The Wheel of Vitality has 12 sections. Look at each section and place a dot on the line marking how satisfied you are with each area of your life. A dot placed at the center of the circle or close to the middle indicates dissatisfaction, while a dot placed on the periphery indicates ultimate happiness.

WHEEL OF VITALITY

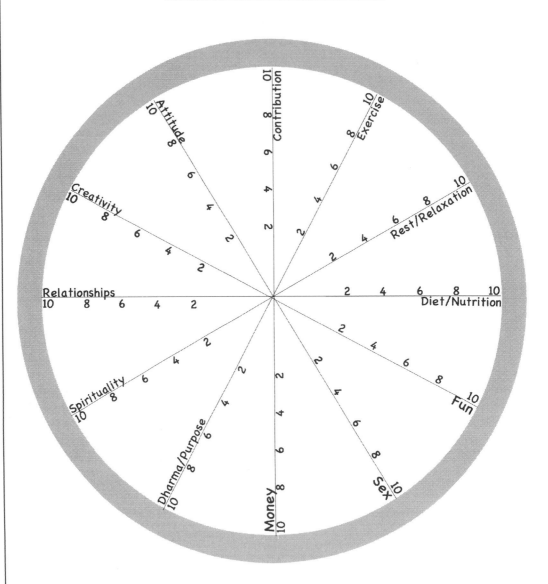

When you have placed a dot on each of the lines, connect the dots to see your circle of life. You will have a clear visual of any imbalances in primary food and a starting point for determining where you may wish to spend more time and energy to create balance and joy in your life.

Goal Setting

Before looking at the food and nutritional information, take a few minutes to set goals. This is an opportunity to establish your health intentions. Take a few moments to write three goals for each time period. They can be simple and basic for now. It is important to begin to think about these things and we will address the "how" over the course of the program.

Today:

Tomorrow:

1 Week:

One month:

Three months:

Six months:

Yogic Principles for Robust Vitality

Over the centuries, yogis have gathered information about the human experience. They have searched, experimented and found ways that are informative, practice and useful. They offer their wisdom to make it easier for us to navigate life.

There are two key concepts from the yogic tradition that provide useful lens for stepping into *robust vitality*. The *chakras*, energetic wheels that are within the body and the *koshas*, sheaths that layer our body. Having these concepts in our tool kit can help navigate the world and give us glimpses into what may be affecting our health and how we can enhance it.

Chakras[2]

In Sanskrit, the word *chakra* is commonly translated to mean "wheel" or "turning." In yogic context, it could also mean "whirlpool" or "vortex." (I find it interesting that the word can be both a noun and a verb — perhaps at the same time.) We can think of the *chakras* as "energy centers" or "globes." These energy centers exist in our "prana" body or "energy suit." In our subtle body, *chakras* represent the intersection of *nadis* (energy) channels — "prana," "qi" or life force flows through these *nadis*. It is useful to think of our *nadis* as roads that lead to the *chakras*, a circle or round about.

Many ancient, Eastern traditions provide interpretations into this *chakra* concept. The Hindu and Buddhist Tantric systems explain the *chakra* system mainly through the central channel of the body (*sushumna*). They see energy flowing from this central channel outward into the rest of the body. Qi Gong has a similar model in which gateways of energy run up and down the central channel and are circulated through meridians (*nadis*). The Bon tradition suggests that the *chakras* have a direct relationship with the quality of our experience. Native Americans

---

2   These materials come from a wide range of sources including: lectures offered from various yoga teachers: Don Stapleton, Naime Jezzeny, Cheryl Crawford, Michael Buck; online sources: wikipedia.com, mindbodygreen.com, chopra.com, chakraenergy.com; and personal experience

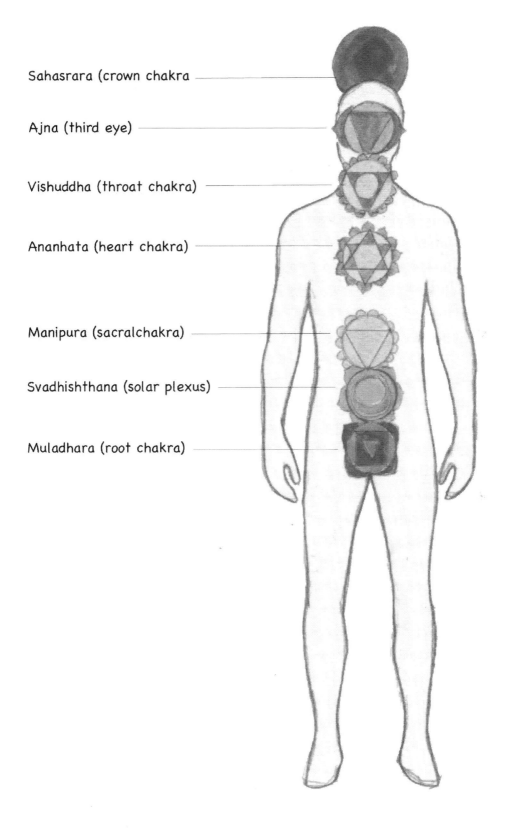

Sahasrara (crown chakra

Ajna (third eye)

Vishuddha (throat chakra)

Ananhata (heart chakra)

Manipura (sacralchakra)

Svadhishthana (solar plexus)

Muladhara (root chakra)

also believe in energy centers and patterns that are relatable to the Hindu *chakra* system.

Western traditions and modern philosophies have adopted these explanations while adding texture and color to the *chakras*. Some even believe that the *chakras* correspond to certain endocrine glands and parts of the nervous system. When the *chakras* are clean, clear and flowing without obstruction, our overall health is vibrant and balanced.

For our purposes we will use the commonly accepted model of the seven *chakra* system which runs up and down the central channel of the body.

1) Muladhara: Root Chakra – *Foundation/Feeling Grounded*
  Location: Base of the Spine
  Color: Red
  Significance: Instinct, Security, Survival (Money and Food),
    Human Potential, Sexuality
  Seed Mantra: Lam

2) Svadhishthana: Sacral Chakra – *Relationship to others and New Experiences*
  Location: Sacrum
  Color: Orange
  Significance: Relationships, Basic Emotional Needs, Pleasure,
    Creativity
  Seed Mantra: Vvam

3) Manipura: Solar Plexus Chakra – *Confidence/Control over our own life*
  Location: Solar Plexus
  Color: Yellow
  Significance: Personal Power, Fear, Anxiety, Transition from
    Simple Emotions to More Complex, Expansiveness, Growth,
    Digestion, Self-worth, Self-esteem
  Seed Mantra: Ram

4) Anahata: Heart Chakra – *Ability to love*
  Location: Heart Center/Chest

Color: Green

Significance: Emotion, Compassion, Equilibrium, Unconditional
    Love, Rejection, Well-being, Passion, Devotion, Circulation,
    Inner Peace

Seed Mantra: Yam

5) Vishuddha: Throat Chakra – *Communication*

Location: Throat

Color: Blue

Significance: Communication, Independence, Security, Fluent
    Thought, Self-Expression

Seed Mantra: Ham

6) Ajna: Third Eye Chakra – *Vision/Seeing the big picture*

Location: Middle of Forehead

Color: Violet

Significance: Balancing Higher and Lower Self, Trusting Inner
Guidance, Intuition, Visual Consciousness, Decision Making

Seed Mantra: Aum

7) Sahasrara: Crown Chakra – *Connection with Spirit*

Location: Above the Head

Color: White

Significance: Unity, Universal Consciousness, Meditation, Inner
Wisdom, State of Pure Consciousness

Seed Mantra: Sound of the Spheres, Silence

Koshas

One of the ways yogis describe the human experience is through
the *koshas*, sheaths or layers. Many believe that there are five layers
contained within each other, like Russian dolls. These layers cover every
aspect of our being, from the most subtle to the most gross and all are
interacting with each other at all times. Whatever we do has an effect
on all layers, an effect on our overall way of being. This is a conceptual
model of looking at reality; yet one that can provide insight on our quest
for *robust vitality*.

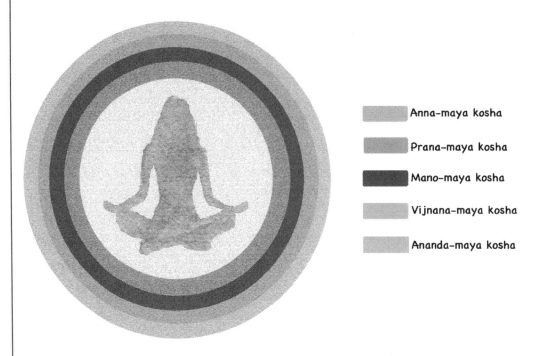

Anna-maya kosha

Prana-maya kosha

Mano-maya kosha

Vijnana-maya kosha

Ananda-maya kosha

1) Annamaya Kosha — *Physical Body/Food Body*

This is our physical body — all the muscles, bones, organs, cells, blood, etc. This *kosha* is typically the one that most of us are concerned with when it comes to our appearance, how we feel and how well we are functioning. This is the body that we suffer when it's sick and enjoy when it is thriving. Many of the food and health concepts in *Robust Vitality* are geared toward enhancing and maintaining this kosha.

2) Pranamaya Kosha — *Energy Body*

The Chinese call it *chi*; the yogis call it *prana*; and in the West we call it energy. This has to do with how energy flows through our bodies. Diet and exercise are two components of keeping our energy flowing. Breathing is another key aspect to maintaining a healthy energy body. This *kosha* is important when we are moving from illness back into health.

3) Manomaya Kosha — *Mental Body*

This *kosha* is our state of thinking. If we are concerned or stressed about something, it tends to live in the *manomaya kosha*. Over-thinking, worry and mental stress are all parts of this *kosha*. In the West we have a tendency to spend a lot of time in this *kosha*. Alternate Nostril

Breathing and the meditations provided can help us bring balance and calm to this *kosha*.

4) Vijnamaya Kosha — *Intuition Body*

This is the *kosha* where we find intuition, innate wisdom and access to greater knowledge. It is through this *kosha* that we begin to connect with something greater than ourselves. We feel supported by unseen forces and part of life's "flow" when we integrate and harmonize with the *vijnamaya kosha*. Move beyond survival and security and into compassion, love and joy. Find harmony in physical body, fluidity in our energy body and stress free in our mental body.

5) Anandamaya Kosha — *Bliss Body*

Yogis consider this bliss body a full connection to spirit. This is where and how we connect with feelings of a nondual, unabiding space of pure joy and bliss. It may seem like this *kosha* is impossible to attain or something rather fantasmigorical; but it is a potential which we can enthusiastically pursue.

Investigate

A self-evaluation can give you a starting point for where you are in your process of purification. The questionnaire below comes from the book, *The Detox Prescription* by Woodson Merrell, M.D. This evaluation will give you a general understanding of your physical and emotional status.

DIRECTIONS:

Answer each question on a scale from 0-4

    0 = I never experience this symptom

    1 = I occasionally experience this symptom, but its not severe

    2 = I occasionally experience this symptom, and it's severe

    3 = I often experience this symptom, but its not severe

    4 = I often experience this symptom and its severe

Head:

Do you have headaches?____

Do you feel faint?____

Do you feel dizzy?____

Do you suffer from insomnia?____

Sub Total _____

Digestion:

Do you feel nauseous or have bouts of vomiting?____

Do you have diarrhea?____

Do you have constipation?____

Do you frequently burp or pass gas?____

Do you feel bloated?____

Sub Total _____

Muscle and Joints:

Do you have pain or aches in your joints?____

Do you have arthritis?____

Do you feel stiff or feel limited in your movements?____

Are your muscles stiff, painful or achy?____

Do you feel physically weak?____

Sub Total _____

Eating and Weight:

Do you indulge in binge eating or drinking?____

Do you crave particular foods?____

Are you overweight?____

Are you underweight?____

Do you retain water?____

Do you eat compulsively or mindlessly?____

Sub Total _____

Energy Level:

Do you feel fatigued or sluggish?____

Do you feel apathetic or lethargic?____

Do you feel hyperactive?____

Do you feel restless?____

Sub Total _____

Mind:

Is your memory short or faulty?_____

Do you have trouble comprehending information?_____

Are you uncoordinated?_____

Do you find it difficult to make decisions?_____

Do you stutter or stammer?_____

Do you slur your speech?_____

Do you suffer from a learning disability?_____

Sub Total _____

Emotions:

Do you have mood swings?_____

Are you anxious, fearful, or nervous?_____

Are you angry, aggressive or irritable?_____

Are you depressed?_____

Sub Total _____

Eyes:

Are your eyes itchy or irritated?_____

Are you eyelids swollen, sticky or red?_____

Do you have bags or dark circles under your eyes?_____

Do you have blurry or tunnel vision?_____

Sub Total _____

Ears:
Are your ears itchy on the inside?_____
Do you suffer from earaches or infections?_____
Do you experience ringing in your ears?_____
Do you have drainage from your ears?_____
Sub Total _____

Nose:
Do you have stuffy nose?_____
Do you have sinus problems?_____
Do you suffer from hay fever?_____
Do you have sneezing attacks?_____
Do you have excessive mucus formation?_____
Sub Total _____

Mouth and Throat:
Do you have a chronic cough?_____
Do you frequently feel the need to clear your throat?_____
Do you have a sore throat, hoarseness, or loss of voice?_____
Are your lips, tongue, or gums swollen or discolored?_____
Sub Total _____

Skin:
Do you have acne?_____
Do you get hives, rashes, or patches of dry skin?_____
Do you have hair loss?_____
Do you suffer from flushing or hot flashes?_____
Are you excessively sweaty?_____
Sub Total _____

Heart Health:
Do you ever experience irregular or skipped heart beat?_____
Do you ever experience rapid or pounding heartbeats?_____
Do you ever experience chest pain?_____
Sub Total _____

Respiratory System:

    Do you have chest congestion?_____

    Do you suffer from asthma or bronchitis?_____

    Do you have shortness of breath?_____

    Do you have difficulty breathing?_____

                                Sub Total _____

General Health:

    Do you get sick frequently?_____

    Do you feel the need to urinate urgently or frequently?_____

    Do you suffer from genital itch or discharge?_____

                                Sub Total _____

GRAND TOTAL _____

0-50 Keep it clean. Everything is fine; a detox plan is not urgently needed.

50-70 Toxins on board. You are just starting to see the effects of accumulated toxins, undertaking a cleanse will be a real lifesaver for you. The sooner you start- the sooner you will see the results. At this stage you truly can be your own best physician.

70-100 Take actions now. Significant diagnosis, high blood pressure, sugar, high cholesterol, its essential to do a cleanse now.

100 and above, 911. You need to seek medical attention, find an expert in functional medicine, do not just do a juice cleanse, do a combined juice and pH diet food program.

Chapter 2

Space

Between stimulus and response there is a space.
In that space is our power to choose our response.
In our response lies our growth and our freedom.
—Viktor Frankl

Sacred Space

Sacred space, is a state of being, a physical place, consciousness and a safe environment. In it, one or many people, spirits and personalities intermingle in ways that are exploratory and developmental. During your reading and experimentation numerous things will surface that can be processed. Experiences from our "multi-dimensional self" will arise in ways that can be colorful and soft, explosive and scary, beautiful, mysterious and enlightening. Old unresolved issues may rise from former burial sites that can be life-affirming and life-enhancing.

Respecting yourself (and others) during this process is necessary and essential. Being nonjudgmental is a key aspect of holding and creating sacred space. It frees oneself from the shackles of life's dualities, which allows for personal unification and harmony. As an individual (and as a community), it is necessary that we maintain a compassionate nonjudgmental attitude as we integrate our *stuff*.

"We don't know what we don't know" is a phrase often used by my teacher Don Stapleton, Ph.D. to describe the learning and developmental process. As the unknown becomes known it is important to appreciate everything revealed. He also likes to say, "it takes the time it takes." This is important to remember as we dive into our own personal sacred being. Allow yourself as much time, in as much (sacred) space to integrate your experience.

Sacred Space is dynamic and not limited to physical space; yet, in this section, we will specifically focus on physical space. We will review and explore how to create a physical sacred space; so that we may have a safe environment to work through our physical, mental and emotional *stuff*.

Types of Space

Home Environment

Our physical space includes our house, car, office or hotel room — anywhere that we stake claim in any sort of way for as little as a few moments. For a yogi, their mat is sacred space. For travelers, it could be their backpack, tent or hotel room. Begin to take note of your surroundings and start to see things as sacred, as yours and as living breathing extensions of yourself.

Consider the *feeling* of your home. Is it inviting? Are you happy to be in it? Does it invite others? Are the walls the colors you want? Is the furniture the right size? This place is where you occupy your corner of the world — what sort of feeling does it provide for you when you think about it?

Essential Locations

Kitchen: A good place to start is your kitchen. It is the place where you feed and sustain your body. Keep it clean and organized. Notice what is in your cupboards, the usefulness of your appliances and what is on your counters. How are they contributing or detracting from your physical goals? What can be thrown out, replaced or organized?

Bedroom: Another place in your home to focus is your bedroom. This is the place where you recharge. It is your sanctuary of serenity. Keep your bed made and closets organized. Make it an inviting environment to rest deeply.

Vehicle: Consider your car. Your car is your vehicle, your transport, your chariot. It brings you to that important meeting, to the date with a friend or lover, to the airport or wherever you need to go. Get it washed, keep it vacuumed and get the oil changed. These observances are not just a list of chores, they are 'the Buddha asking us to pay attention' as one of my teachers says.

Office: Imagine your office. Does it inspire creativity? Is it a place that attracts abundance? Does it have personality? Your workplace, whether it be an office, studio, classroom or field, can add or detract to the value of your life. Does it look and feel that way when it comes to mind? Is it ideal for generating prosperity?

Another important point to note is that your office typically is the place for filing and storing important documents. These documents realistically represent a connection with your income. So, keep your records filed and organized and get rid of any of the old stuff. Old credit card bills, insurance records and any extraneous outdated information can decrease your chances for achieving your optimum financial goals. Consider this a worthy step in reaching your wealth goals. What are your wealth goals? Is this the sort of place that helps you achieve them?

Electronic Space

In our modern era, we are constantly bombarded with electro-magnetic fields (EMFs). Studies are showing that EMFs can be detrimental: fatigue, dizziness, nausea and even greater diseases are being linked to EMF exposure. Be mindful of how much time you spend on or in front of electronic devices. Take some time to protect yourself using EMF blockers for your body, computer and entire house. Two useful websites are:

1. http://www.safespaceprotection.com

2. http://www.blockemf.com

Your computer hard-drive, email, smart phone, and social networking outlets can all get overrun with communications and information. These technologies can leave you feeling overwhelmed and stuck. Take time to sort through, organize and delete daily.

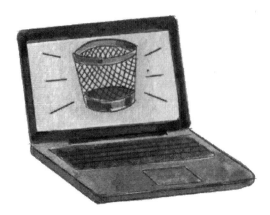

On your computer spend some time to organize the pictures from your last vacation into a slide show. Delete old stored documents that no longer have relevance. Emails can become overwhelming if we have too much junk in our boxes. Just like physical junk mail, throw it out, unsubscribe, or trash it. If something really strikes you as important, file it in a folder or respond to it. An overflowing email box is often a burden and can create 'inbox anxiety.' Get rid of a couple at a time; and before you know it, you will look forward to seeing what comes in. Looking forward and being excited about things is the exact sort of energy that will be returned to you if that is what you are producing. Frustration, irritation and fatigue will be returned if that is how you are spending your time. How can you organize to make your electronic life more exciting?

There are two programs that I use on my computer to eliminate advertisements and pop-ups. Since doing this I have noticed increased clarity and focus when I surf the net. They are both free to download:

1. Ghostery: https://www.ghostery.com/en/

2. Adblock Plus (ABP): https://adblockplus.org

Mental & Emotional Space

Mental/emotional clearing can be the most challenging and the scariest form of clearing — but it does not have to be. By the time you have de-cluttered, you will have actually worked on much of the mental/emotional components of yourself. Your stuff and your physical body are outer manifestations of your mental/emotional states. By de-cluttering your space you have invited fresh and creative energy into your life. By organizing your photo albums you have begun to address any unlocked emotions.

There are many ways to address mental/emotional work and by no means is this a small task. Author Jed McKenna suggests a process that he calls "spiritual autolysis." Even though his process is aimed at enlightenment and finding truth, it healthfully serves our practical pursuits. Instead of searching for truth, he suggests that we shed untruth. He suggests that we begin a process of writing things down until we think we have written something that is authentically true. This is a wonderful process of awareness and is suggested for those that like to write and particularly for those that do not. It unwinds our thoughts, (similar to the *Unwinding Your Day Meditation* offered in the Meditation Section) and reveals the true source of these thoughts.

Another way of looking at this process is as if we are deprogramming ourselves from all the junk that we have collected over the years. Notice what is yours and the many things you've been carrying for/ from other's.

Another way of experimenting with this sort of clearing is becoming aware of our reactions to the people, things and events that happen around us. How do we feel when someone pushes our buttons? When thoughts and emotions emerge, it is an opportunity for us to learn about ourselves. If we do not have any 'buttons that can be pushed' then we can be happy and healthy.

In the affirmation section we explore ways to use our brain to stimulate mental/emotional change. Our minds are like a garden and we must tend to them regularly. Planting, watering and weeding are all parts of this process. What needs to be planted? What needs to be watered? What needs to be pulled? See the discussion on *Vital Nutrients* and the *Quality of Life Inventory* to have a deeper look at these things.

Physical Body

Your physical body needs to be cleared too. One of the keys to optimum health and *robust vitality* is to clear out toxicity. In the cleansing section we discuss ways to do this. It is important to know that good physical health is an important part of our human experience. Outside of our mental/ emotional stressors, 3 main components make physical health: 1) healthful nutritional sources 2) elimination of toxicity 3) exercise. Clear space in your body to make space in your heart.

The Importance of Clearing Clutter

Diets, cleanses, and physical exercise are usually what we think of when it comes to cleansing. Clearly it is important to take care of our physical bodies, but we must not overlook another key component to cleansing — our home environment. Just like your body, your house can become sick, overweight and low energy causing disharmony. Clearing clutter to create *sacred space* is important for our overall health and assimilating any experiences that may be lodged or stuck.

Creating sacred space starts with our personal physical space, which is is a key aspect for *robust vitality*. The art of designing and maintaining a home (or any space we live, work or play in, even if only for a short time) is a practice worth investigating. You are invited to expand your definition of cleansing by practicing the art of creating sacred space. We can enter into a whole new dimension of what it means to be fit, healthy and clean.

Creating sacred space by clearing clutter is more than just a house cleanse, it is an entire mental, emotional, physical and spiritual experience.

The elimination of clutter provides us with the opportunity to invite in a newer, fresher and cleaner energy.

A spiritual teacher introduced me to this practice several years ago. Along with a regiment of daily meditation and bodily cleanses, he suggested clearing clutter. I scoffed and thought: "What is the value in that? Besides, I don't have that much stuff anyway." Like a teenager asked to make his bed, I begrudgingly began this process and found more than I anticipated. Some things were quite easy to toss, while other things I clung to — and they clung to me. Immediately, I could feel the powerful effects of this practice. I was sleeping better, thinking more clearly, had more energy and I even lost some physical weight. My life began to flow with more ease — I was astounded.

It was not all easygoing though. After I cleaned some parts of my closet and attic, I then found letters, pictures and old books. This process became quite intense as my emotions bubbled up. Could I really be holding onto this letter from an old lover? This picture of a traumatic accident, did I really need another painful reminder? Why did I have this book that I never read? They represented and perpetuated blockages in my life and once I released some of them, romance, revitalization and information came flooding my way.

The art of cultivating sacred space became more and more real as I practiced. Cleanliness really was godliness. Less was more. "Purge to merge," my teacher would say. As I took more care and appreciation for my things, I became more appreciative and caring toward myself and others. The practice was so incredibly transformative that it was as if I had undergone years of therapy in a few short months.[1]

Just as we surround ourselves with like-minded and hearted individuals, we also surround ourselves with like-minded and hearted stuff. This stuff, in its raw energetic form is the outward expression of who we are — it mirrors our internal landscape.

---

1 On the popular television show, "Hoarders" a psychologist is brought along to counsel the hoarder. This speaks to the deep levels of mental and emotional disturbance gripping tight to our stuff can have on our psyche.

Karen Kingston, Fueng Shui artist and author writes,[2] "Everything in your outer life - especially your home environment — mirrors your inner self. Conversely, everything in your home has an affect on you, from the smallest object to the largest design structure" (Kingston 11-12).

By diving into the inquiry of our stuff, we can see ourself in new ways. How is your stuff impacting your health? Now is the time to release and recharge. Kingston also suggests that, "when we are out of balance with our surroundings, we become physically, mentally, emotionally, and spiritually sick" (Kingston 16).

By letting go of our stuff we literally 'let go' of *stuff*. Detaching from our things allows us to embrace the notion of nonattachment, a core spiritual concept in many wisdom traditions. Breaking the bondage with material things activates a deeper sense of clarity, calmness and serenity. This allows us to open and explore more deeply the *now* moments.

You don't need to be a spiritual person or have intensive training to create a sacred place. You can create sacred space by consciously decorating — just place everything with intention. Look at it. Feel it. See what it is offering. Consider what value a new thing will provide. Just like the old saying, "if you can't improve upon the silence, don't speak," if you can't improve upon the space, don't fill it. Position things where and how you want them. Remember: Everything has its place and everything in its place.

It might be overwhelming at first to think of all the stuff in your home or office that needs a good "Spring cleaning." Well, this practice is good for all seasons, so take a deep *grounding breath* (p.42-43) and jump right in. Ask yourself: What is it that you are, literally and figuratively, sweeping under the rug? What are you holding on to and, deeper still,

---

2 Her book, *Creating Sacred Space with Feung Shui*, Karen Kingston writes about the "art of living" as being a part of our human experience. Kingston dedicates an entire chapter to the practice of clearing clutter. "Clutter accumulates when energy stagnates. Healthy energy is moving energy" (Kingston 42). Another author who writes about the significance of clearing clutter is Elain St. James. See her book entitled, *Simplify Your Life, 100 Ways to Slow Down and Enjoy the Things that Really Matter*, in which she starts with the reducing clutter.

what is holding on to you? What does it mean to live in a sacred space? This may take some time, so enjoy the process.

Lastly, consider all space sacred.

10 Tips for Clearing Space

1. **Observe:** Observe your environment and notice what you are projecting and what is reflecting back at you. There is a telling dynamic at play. Consider all space sacred and see how your perspective changes. What is impeding or enhancing your journey? What are you great at doing and what are you avoiding? How can you make your space sacred?

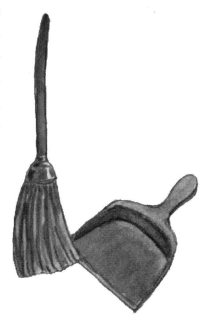

2. **The Story of Your Stuff:** Take a mental/emotional inventory in each room. How does the room make you feel when you first walk in? Is your bedroom inviting you for deep rest and relaxation? Does your kitchen offer your body the nourishment it needs? Is your office a place that will provide you with the clean and precise 'tools of your trade?'

What are the things you notice? How are they arranged? When you look at something, what emotions are stirred? Do you really need that letter from a former partner? Is it useful to have that painting that makes you nervous? Do you feel abundant or anxious when you check your valuables?

The quality of your emotional reaction is more valuable than the thing itself. Investigate your environment and see how it might be impacting your multi-dimensional health. Be curious with your surroundings and explore with childlike vigor.

3. **The 80/20 Rule:** The 80/20 Rule shows that, on average, we use 20% of our stuff 80% of the time. Take this fresh perspective on your things and move slowly to eliminate the 80% of the things you use 20% of the time. This does not mean it all goes right away; the Rule is a guideline for success. Use it as a lens for clearing.

4. **Start Somewhere That Is Easy:** Find a place that you know will be emotionally and physically easy, like your closet. Put on your favorite music, a gentle smile on your face and get to work. Whatever you absolutely love, stays. Whatever you do not goes into 2 possible piles: 1) Discard 2) Maybe. Get rid of the discard pile and reserve the maybe pile to do at a later date. Ask yourself if you really need that old garment or that extra pair of shoes. When was the last time you wore them?

5. **I Can't Remember:** We all have things that we don't know what to do with (the "maybe" pile) or don't remember we even had. Put these things into a box, close it and put it somewhere safe for 6 weeks. If you can't remember what's in it, take the whole box and get rid of it. If you didn't need anything in the box, get rid of it.

6. **The Tougher Stuff:** Pictures, books, letters, paintings and antiques can be particularly difficult to let go of. Consolidate your pictures into a nice album. Read through letters and toss the ones that don't uplift you. Ceremonial fires for letters and significant writings are great ways to clear any old blockages while simultaneously setting ablaze. Check your bookshelf and consider when was the last time you cracked those books. You can always find them at your library, especially if you donate them there.

7. **Where to put it:** There are plenty of services that will come to your house and pick up your stuff, like the Vietnam Veterans Association. It can even be used as a tax right off. Local shopping areas have (clothes) drop off bins. Charity drives are great as well. You can also turn your old stuff into cash. Yard Sales, ebay and consignment stores are available. Set time lines for yourself and if it is not worn, read or shared by a certain date, donate it.

8. **Get Help:** Enlist your kids, spouse or neighbors. Hire a personal organizer. Consider this part of your mental, emotional health care plan. It is worth it – YOU are worth it.

9. **Bring in Plants:** Plants are a great way to spruce up your environment. Fresh flowers make lively additions to any room and potted plants help to purify and circulate the air. They enjoy your singing and classical music is a favorite.

10. **Reward Yourself:** After cleaning an area in your house or office, take a break, smile and breathe in the new freshness of the area. Treat yourself to a movie or a massage. If you do buy something, remember to get rid of at least one, preferably two other things to make space for that newbie.

Create an Altar

An altar is a place that is dedicated for cultivating your spiritual energy. It is a place to inspire and uplift our spirit. It is a place center our energy. It is a place to honor yourself, your life, your dreams, and to salute a higher power. It is a place to offer gratitude, to pray, to meditate and to generate a conscious energy that brings us to higher and deeper levels of fulfillment. It is a place that reminds you that you are magnificent, amazing, joyful and connected to something greater. With all your newly created sacred space, find a special place and make it extra special.

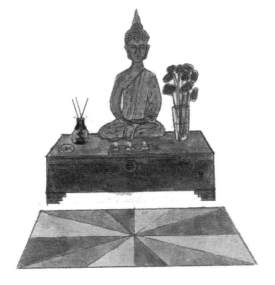

Suggestions For Building An Altar and Maintaining Its Power

a. Clean and organize an area in your personal space. An area that you like and that you can maintain in a way that is extra special. Traditionally these types of altars face East. Try and find an Eastward facing direction, if not, that is ok, but choose the area with intention.

b. Find something that can act as a table or pedestal for your objects. I use an antique wooden box. I have seen some people use small bookshelves or ledges hanging off walls. Some people use coffee tables and others use full-size tables.

c. Lovingly place a few special objects that have specific meaning upon the surface. Pictures of deities or teachers, special stones or seashells, and symbols of financial abundance like a ring or watch are all great things for your altar. Flowers and candles are nice touches as well. Get creative with this, and remember that each object stands for something greater.

d. Place a small prayer rug, cushion or special mat as an invitation for you to join the energy of your altar. The altar is a place to go to as often as you like. Try once a day, and then work toward several times. Morning and evening are good times to check in with your altar.

e. Establish a relationship with your altar as a place to charge your intentions, let go or simply relax. It is a place to ask for guidance and encourage loved ones on their path. It is a place where meditation can take place. It is a place to go inside and notice the stillness within.

f. When the altar is set up, keep it clean and organized. Experiment with the position of the objects until it is just the way you desire. This is a great way to experiment with your intuition and feeling. How does the design and actual placement impact your experience? Does the placement of things even matter?

g. Enjoy the process and enjoy your altar.

Chapter 3

Breathing

The only thing we can control in life is our breath.
—Yogi Bhajan

The Importance of Breathing

We can go weeks to months without food, days without water, but only minutes without oxygen. Many of us take breathing for granted because it is automatic. With a bit of focus, we can become aware of our breathing patterns. By engaging with them we enhance our overall wellbeing.

How aware of your breath are you? When was the last time you counted ten breaths in a row? Have you noticed how your breath changes based on the situation you are in? Watching a scary movie, arguing with someone, love making or while at work, do we have the same type/quality of breath?

By simply paying attention to our breath, we can bring deeper under-standing to what is happening in our internal and external worlds. We have the ability to access our mental, emotional and physical dimensions through breath. Our breath is an indicator of our centeredness, connect-edness and cohesiveness with our multi-dimensionality. They meet at the point of the breath.

Did you know that both anxiety and excitement function the same physiologically? The only thing that may be different is the breath. Did you know that cancer cannot survive in an oxygen rich environment? In fact most diseases cannot. Fear, stress, anxiety and negativity cannot survive in an oxygen rich environment.

In his book, *The Only Answer to Cancer*, Dr. Leonard Coldwell's preferred treatment for cancer is oxygen therapy. Dr. Coldwell refer-ences two of his predecessors:

Since Nobel Prize winner Otto Warburg has scientifically proven that cancer cells cannot grow or exist in an oxygen rich environment or an alkaline environment as proved by Nobel Prize winner Max Plank, it is very simple and easy to understand that by creating oxygen-rich and slightly alkaline body environment, the cancers cells have to disappear (Coldwell 38).

One of the most powerful disease prevention and treatment methods is simple, natural and free: breathing. So, explore your breath. Discover the strength and efficacy behind breath practice.

Listed below are five different techniques to forge a deeper relation-ship with our breath. Many of the practices come out of yogic traditions, but are all not limited to yogis nor are they designed with any religious or philosophical intent. They are meant to enhance our body's experi-ence with itself.

Techniques
Belly and Heart Breathing

1) Become aware of your breath without trying to change it.
   Notice its:
   - quality
   - texture
   - sound

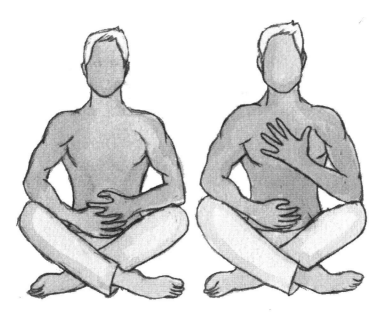

- length of inhalations and exhalations

Observe:

- the rise and fall of your chest
- the expansion and contraction of your rib cage
- any movement in your belly or elsewhere in your body

Allow your consciousness to float upon your breath like a leaf on a stream.

2) Place one hand on your belly and one hand on your heart. With your focus and intention breathe through your nose into your hands. Allow your belly to expand and contract, rise and fall. Allow your ribs and chest to expand.

3) Exhale through your nose slowly and visualize the breath going out.

It's as simple as that.

Review:

- Notice your breath.
- Breathe in and out through your nose.
- One hand on your belly and the other hand on your heart.
- Inhale into your hands filling the belly and chest.
- Exhale slowly through your nose.

Do this for 5 minutes per day.

Grounding Breath

The Grounding Breath is used when you are feeling unsettled or after an intense experience or physical practice. I often employ this technique before and after examinations, presentations and lectures. One of my yoga teachers has us do this before class and another after class, try both. After long flights or car trips this technique can also be very helpful – the benefits are astounding. Try it and enjoy the benefits.

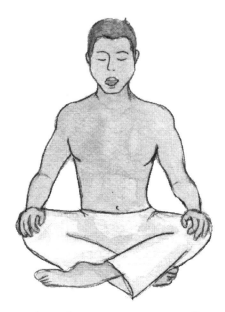

1. Take note of your breath. Become aware of it without trying to change it. Notice its quality, texture, sound, length of inhalations and exhalations. Observe the rise and fall of your chest, the expansion and contraction of your rib cage and any movement in your belly or elsewhere in your body. Allow your consciousness to float upon your breath like a leaf on a stream, buoyantly coasting along.

2. Inhale through nose and allow the exhalation to exit through the mouth. On the out breath, if there is more air left in your lungs, let it out.

3. On the next inhalation begin the breath by visualizing it starting from your feet and moving up to the top of your head. Allow the exhale to happen through the mouth, visualizing it coming from the top of your head exiting out through your feet.

4. The next inhalation will happen naturally without having to think about it. Bring your mindfulness back to your feet and inhale from the tips of your toes all the way to the top of your head. This time allow your shoulders to lift up as you inhale. Upon exhaling, allow your shoulders to drop with gravity. Feel the out breath leave from the top of your head through your fingertips and toes.

5. Make a conscious effort to connect to the earth with every exhalation.

Alternate Nostril Breathing – Anuloma Viloma

Alternate Nostril Breathing (known as Anuloma Viloma in Sanskrit) is a great exercise for centering. It helps to balance the hemispheres of the brain creating a greater sense of clarity, focus and mental sharpness. By enhancing the communication between the left and right hemispheres of the brain, our overall sense of physical, mental and psychic well-being are attuned and increased.

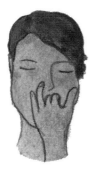 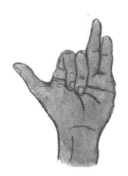 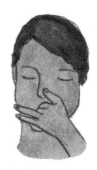

Note: This exercise uses a hand mudra called the Vishnu mudra. Taking our "peace fingers," the index finger and middle finger, folding them into the center of the palm, forms this mudra. The thumb, the ring and pinky finger are extended. Tradition informs us that we are to use our right hand for this mudra. For the sake of upholding tradition begin with your right hand. I see neither difference nor detriment to using your left hand and I often switch hands during this technique.

1. Take note of your breath. Become aware of it without trying to change it. Notice its quality, texture, sound, length of inhalations and exhalations. Observe the rise and fall of your chest, the expansion and contraction of your rib cage and any movement in your belly or elsewhere in your body. Allow your consciousness to float upon your breath like a leaf on a stream, buoyantly coasting along.

2. Take your thumb, push the right nostril closed and exhale slowly out the left nostril (mouth remains closed during the entire exercise).

3. Inhale through the left nostril while maintaining the thumb on the right nostril. Move the index and pinky finger to close the left nostril. Your hand is gently pinching both nostrils shut. Temporarily hold your breath and without straining release the thumb, and exhale out the right nostril (maintain the left nostril closed). Make this a long slow exhalation.

4. Inhale through the right nostril, pinch both nostrils shut, and then release the pinky and index finger exhaling through the left nostril.

5. Go back and forth between nostrils with this exercise for a designated set of breaths. 7, 11, 18, 21, whatever you choose, but make sure to designate a number.

6. To finish take one full breath in and out, close your eyes and feel the effects.

To refine this exercise you can count 4 seconds on the inhale, hold the breath for 4 seconds, exhale for 8 seconds and hold the breath out for 4 seconds, then begin again. There are many versions to this breath but do what feels best for you. If you do not like counting, inhale gently until full, hold your breath for as long as you are comfortable, exhale long slow and controlled, then hold the breath just a bit when fully empty.

Breath of Youth

This breath comes out of the Yoga Tradition. I've learned it in various forms from different teachers. Mietek Wirkus, one of the world's greatest bioenergy healers, taught this particular method to me. He learned it from a Tibetan monk. According to the monk everyone who practices it will experience eternal youth, be able to sense and feel energy transference and protect themselves energetically from others.

1) Become aware of your breath without trying to change it.

   Notice its:
   - quality
   - texture
   - sound
   - length of inhalations and exhalations

   Observe:
   - the rise and fall of your chest
   - the expansion and contraction of your rib cage
   - any movement in your belly or elsewhere in your body

   Allow your consciousness to float upon your breath like a leaf on a stream.

2) Visualize your breath traveling from the base of your spine (pelvis area) up your spine and into your head on an inhalation.

3) Pause gently when your breath comes to your head and image it traveling from the back of your head out your forehead through the center of your brow point (in between your eyes).

4) On the exhalation visualize your breath traveling down the outside of your body (about 4 inches from your body) parallel with your spine.

5) At the bottom of your exhalation pause gently and visualize the breath coming back into the base of your spine around your pelvis area.

6) Inhale and repeat the process.

Now that you have the loop in your mind and your breath following that pattern you will add in a specific count.

Inhale: 8 seconds, the breath moves up the spine.

Pause: 4 seconds, the breath moves from the back of your head out the front of your forehead (about 4 inches outside of your body).

Exhale: 8 seconds, the breath travels down the front of your body
Pause: 4 seconds, the breath travels from outside of your body into
the base of your pelvis.
This type of breathing creates a loop (see diagram).

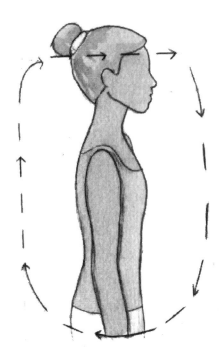

Breath of Fire – Kapalabhati

Kapalabhati means shiny skull or to shine/polish the skull. In Sanskrit:
kapala = skull, bhati = shine. This breath has the ability to awaken the
mind and body, stimulate the digestion, and increase circulation. Certain
monks are known to do Kapalabhati breath as one of their morning
practices. It is a technique that involves short, active exhales and longer
passive inhales.

1. Take note of your breath. Become aware of it without trying to
   change it. Notice its quality, texture, sound, length of inhalations and exhalations. Observe the rise and fall of your chest, the
   expansion and contraction of your rib cage and any movement in
   your belly or elsewhere in your body. Allow your consciousness to
   float upon your breath like a leaf on a stream, buoyantly coasting
   along.

2. To find the location for the action of this breath, take three fingers and place them below the belly button. If you do not have the muscle control for moving your belly, you can push in using your hands. Soon you will be able to do this with just your belly.

3. Quickly contract your belly, forcefully expelling all of the air out of your lungs through your nose (keep your mouth shut).

4. Release the contraction and allow the air to be sucked back into your lungs through your nose. Go slowly at first, and then increase the pace. Start off with 20 repetitions. Eventually you will work up to two sets of 500 with a 1-minute rest in between.

5. To get to 500 repetitions 2 times, start with:
   50 breaths, 1 minute normal breathing, 50 breaths for 1 week
   100 breaths,1 minute normal breathing, 100 breaths for 1 week
   200 breaths, 1 minute normal breathing, 200 breaths for 2 weeks
   300 breaths, 1 minute normal breathing, 300 breaths for 2 weeks
   400 breaths, 1 minute normal breathing, 400 breaths for 2 weeks
   500 breaths, 1 minute normal breathing, 500 breaths

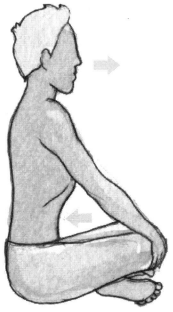

Consciously pull in navel
Sharp exhale trhough nose

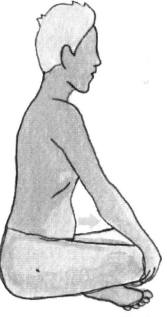

Inhale happens automatically
Navel releases

Chapter 4

Food & Health

The first wealth is health.
—Ralph Waldo Emerson

It goes without saying that eating well is essential for a healthy body. By being mindful of our food choices and staying hydrated, we can ensure that we get the appropriate amount of nutrition. The amount of water we drink, the types of foods we eat, how much we eat, when and where all factor into our overall wellbeing. Conversely, how we are feeling also factors into our food and drink choices. But what does eating well really mean?

What do you choose to eat and drink on a daily basis? Have you read about nutrition or contacted a specialist? What types of snacks do you eat? Have you considered body purification or detoxification? Have you considered the environmental or political impact of your food choices? Have you looked into eating methods, such as chewing, culinary preparation and saying prayers before or after meals?

Our diet and attention to its components are key to being a conscientious eater and a conscious earthling. I suggest we look at the model offered thousands of years ago by Hippocrates, "let food be thy medicine and medicine be thy food." Many consider him to be the father of holistic medicine and his philosophy has been refined with great success many times since.

One notable proponent was Dr. Max Gerson[1] who published a book *A Cancer Therapy: Results of 50 Cases*. He documented successful treatments of cancer (and many other degenerative diseases) using fresh vegetable juices, high alkaline foods, enemas and vitamin supplementation. His daughter Charlotte, who has a nonprofit center in San Diego, CA and two very successful treatment centers located in Mexico and Hungary, continues his work. Even though his practices have been outlawed in the US, the body of healing work that he has created is irrefutable.

The recognition of food and herb based healing methods is gaining popularity in the US. More and more people are exploring natural remedies and experiencing tremendous results. It is wise to supplement any traditional Western treatment with a healthy diet.

Dr. Charles Mayo, the founder of the world famous Mayo Clinic expresses similar sentiments:

> *Here let me repeat one solemn truth which should be repeated over and over each day until everybody comprehends its meaning and acts upon it. Normal resistance to disease is directly dependent upon adequate food. Normal resistance to disease never comes out of pillboxes. Adequate food is the cradle of normal resistance, the playground of normal immunity, the workshop of good health, and the laboratory of long life (emphasis from author).*

In the United States, chronic diseases, cancer, diabetes and obesity are all on the rise. According to the American Cancer Society it is estimated that there were 1,665,540 new cancer cases diagnosed and 585,720 cancer deaths in the US in 2014. Cancer remains the second most common cause of death in the US, accounting for nearly 1 of every 4 deaths.[2] Diabetes has been rising at about 8% each year and costs the

---

1 Visit www.gerson.org for more information.

2 http://www.cancer.org/research/cancerfactsstatistics/cancerfactsfigures2014/index

country $245 million dollars in 2012.[3] Almost 2 million new cases were diagnosed for ages 20 and older in 2010.[4]

Some of this has to do with toxicity, yet much of it is due to poor food choices, which can lead to obesity. According to the Center of Disease Control and Prevention, more than one-third of U.S. adults (35.7%) are obese. Obesity-related conditions include heart disease, stroke, Type 2 Diabetes and certain types of cancer which are some of the leading causes of preventable death.[5] Obesity is an easily curable disease — we have the power to improve our diets and heal ourselves.

Unfortunately, the mainstream answer to many of these health issues is to medicate. Just pop a pill. The percentage of people using at least one prescription drug in the past month is 48.5% (2007-2010).[6] Prescription drugs kill more people annually than illegal drugs. There has been a 300% rise in prescription drug related deaths since 1990.[7] These deaths and diseases are preventable.

According to the CDC, "from 2000 to 2015 more than half a million people died from drug overdoses. 91 Americans die every day from an opioid overdose."[8]

Dr. Bruce Lipton, in his book *The Biology of Belief*, shares his sentiments about prescription drugs, "Using prescription drugs to silence a body's symptoms enables us to ignore personal involvement we may have with the onset of these symptoms. The overuse of prescription drugs provides a vacation from personal responsibility" (Lipton p.82). By taking responsibility, we have the power to cure our bodies and reverse

---

3 http://www.cnn.com/2013/03/06/health/diabetes-cost-report/ and http://www.cdc.gov/mmwr/preview/mmwrhtml/mm6145a4.htm

4 http://www.diabetes.org/diabetes-basics/statistics/

5 http://www.cdc.gov/obesity/data/adult.html The estimated annual medical cost of obesity in the U.S. was $147 billion in 2008 U.S. dollars; the medical costs for people who are obese were $1,429 higher than those of normal weight

6 http://www.cdc.gov/nchs/fastats/drugs.htm Percent of persons using three or more prescription drugs in the past month: 21.7% (2007-2010) Percent of persons using five or more prescription drugs in the past month: 10.6% (2007-2010)

7 http://www.cdc.gov/homeandrecreationalsafety/rxbrief/

8 https://www.cdc.gov/drugoverdose/epidemic/index.html

these trends by making better food choices, detoxifying and exercising.

This next section will explore some basic concepts involving food and nutrition to establish healthy lifestyle choices. These principles are useful guidelines for maximizing physical health. There is always more information available, so check the suggested reading list if one or any of these categories peaks your interest and appetite.

Basic Concepts
Alkaline Food[9]

An acid/alkaline balanced diet is a diet that facilitates optimum pH levels in your body for the digestion and absorption of nutrients. Acidic foods, when digested by your body, produce toxic waste, whereas alkaline foods leave vitamins, minerals and nutrients for your body to use. Calcium, magnesium, iron and copper are left by alkaline foods, all of which neutralize the acidic effects on your body. When these minerals are *not* present, acidosis occurs which can permeate your blood stream and organs leaving a platform for disease. By consuming alkaline foods and beverages much of the damage caused by acidosis can be reversed.

A Bit of Chemistry

PH stands for "potential of hydrogen" and measures the acidic/alkaline level of something. A pH of 0 is totally acidic, while a pH of 14 is completely alkaline. A pH of 7 is neutral. These levels vary throughout your body and throughout the course of the day. Your blood is slightly alkaline, with a pH between 7.35 and 7.45. Your stomach is very acidic, with a pH of 3.5 or below, so it can break down food. And your urine changes, depending on what you eat — that's how your body keeps the level in your blood steady.

A normal body fluctuates between 7.35 and 7.45 for pH. This promotes healthy digestion, mineral absorption, cell repair and energy levels.

---

9 Useful Websites: http://www.acetoacetanilide.net
http://www.dummies.com/how-to/content/acid-alkaline-diet-for-dummies-cheat-sheet.
html http://health.usneas.com/best-diet/acid-alkaline-diet

Dangers of Acidosis

The Standard American Diet (S.A.D.) is highly acidic because it contains large amounts of refined grains, animal products, processed foods and sugar (along with all the "avoids"). An acidified body is deprived of oxygen and vital nutrients to support your body's functions. Your body must leach vitamins, minerals and enzymes to neutralize the acidosis. Calcium, for example, is one such nutrient that is sequestered from your bones and cells to balance the body's pH. They snatch nutrients like magnesium which aids in calcium absorption, promotes muscle growth and hormone regulation. Besides your teeth and bones, your body will mine these nutrients from organs and tissues as well. Hence the trend of osteoporosis, tooth decay and organ/ tissue damage.

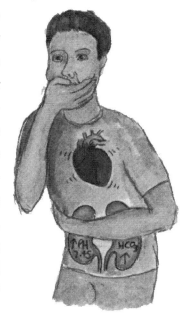

Symptoms of acidosis: joint pain, fatigue, headaches, anxiety, congestion and heartburn.

Everything from a runny nose to skin eruptions, heartburn, eczema, inflammation, arthritis, poor circulation, chronic fatigue, irritable bowel syndrome, a weakened immune system — even cancer — can be traced back in some way to an acidic inner terrain. (*Crazy Sexy Diet* p. 23)

Are you experiencing any of these symptoms with regularity? Just because you may not be experiencing these symptoms, or not recognizing them, does not mean that you do not have some level of acidosis.

What Foods Are Alkaline And What Are Acidic?

In general, fresh fruits and vegetables are alkaline. The more you cook or process them the more they turn into acidic foods. For example red peppers are a great alkalizing food in their raw state, but once cooked they become highly acidic.

Acidic foods are most animal products: meat, fish, milk, eggs, cheese, poultry as well as grains, sugar and pasta. We must include processed food products in this category as well. Anything that comes in a plastic wrapper or packaging, with the exception of fresh items, is generally acidic and typically toxic.

Dr. Robert Young in his book *The pH Miracle* states, "striking the optimum 80/20 balance can result in dramatic weight loss, rebuilt stamina... and vibrant health" (Silberstein p. 28). The 80/20 rule = 80% plants, 20% animal foods. This correlates to roughly 80% alkaline and 20% acidic. Strive toward an 80/20 balance of alkaline to acid foods.

To test your pH, you can purchase urine strips that will give you a good indicator of your levels. Do not take your first urination of the day and be mindful that depending on what and when you eat, your test results may vary.

Enzymes

What Are Enzymes And What To They Do?

The word enzyme comes from the Greek language, meaning, "to ferment," or "cause a change." Enzymes are catalysts that help encourage digestive and metabolic processes — they are the life force generating these processes. Quality of life is directly proportionate to amount of available enzymes. In fact, the miracle of life would be impossible without enzymes.

According to Dr. Edward Howell, father of modern enzyme therapy, enzymes are the body's workers. Enzymes are catalysts for biological and chemical reactions in the body: they help repair DNA and RNA; they help transform and store energy; they make hormones, dissolve fiber and prevent clotting, and inflammation; they balance and enhance immune system; they can help to heal things like cancer, arthritis, diabetes, digestive issues, obesity, high-cholesterol.[10] They also play an important role in the detoxification process.

---

10 *Rainbow Green Live-Food Cuisine*, Dr. Gabriel Cousens p. 112-113 *Conscious Eating*, Dr. Gabriel Cousens p. 523-536

Essentially, they help build, restore, repair and maintain our bodies. Everything from digestion to blinking our eyes is the result of an enzymatic process. "Every cell in the body produces enzymes which are used to power physical movements, regulate organ function and power the immune system."[11] Enzyme and enzyme production is a key component for healthful living and longevity.

The Bank Metaphor

Imagine your body's store of enzymes like a bank account. Our enzyme bank is equivalent to our life force potential. Every time we eat "live," seasonal and organic food, we add to our bank account. Every time we consume lifeless, enzymatic deficient foods, e.g. processed food, hydrogenated oils and sugar we must draw from our bank account.

Along with digesting food we use enzymes to repair, rebuild and restore our body's natural functions, hence making other withdrawals (especially when we are sick). It is as if your maintenance bills are coming due and your bank account is depleted because of unnecessary withdrawals. We now must borrow to provide ourselves with energy. We borrow from stimulants such as caffeine and from our organs and bones, depleting us even further.

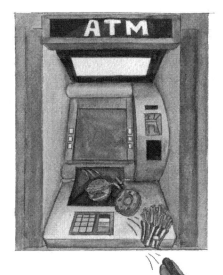

11 *Survival in the 21st Century*, Viktoras Kulvinskas

We need to make health enzyme deposits as regularly as possible so we can thrive in healthy physical abundance. Eating enzyme rich foods, taking supplements and de-stressing are keys to growing our account.

Enzyme Depletion

With stress, age and after illnesses our enzymes decrease. Cooking at boiling point for more than 3 minutes kills all enzymes. The use of pesticides, irradiation and microwaving food decreases the quantity and quality of usable enzymes.

Incomplete digestion from dense foods like dairy and animal protein put a strain on the digestive system (borrowing enzymes) and our immune system. Cooked protein is the most difficult for our body to digest, often causing intestinal toxemia and enzyme depletion. Since our body is unable to assimilate much of this food, it must derive its energy from the organism itself, taxing its enzyme reserves. As Viktoras Kulvinskas points out, "the body must literally consume itself in order to continue to function."[12]

Ways to Increase Enzymes

Eating live, raw foods is the best way to preserve enzymes and maximize health.[13] Not overeating is another way to conserve enzymes. Paavo Airola suggests that not overeating is the most important health and longevity secret.[14] In Okinawa, Japan they eat slowly and deliberately until they are 80% full. Smaller plates and extra chewing will help with portion control.

Plant based digestive enzymes are the most bio-available source of enzymes. This means that by eating vegetables, we can access the most efficient source of enzymes.

According to Dr. John Douillard, a congested bile duct can block flow of digestive enzymes. Remember those dense protein sources?

---

12 *Survival in the 21ˢᵗ Century*

13 *Conscious Eating*, Dr. Cousens p.528

14 *Conscious Eating*, Dr. Cousens p.529

They stress the liver and can contribute to sludgy bile. Dr. Douillard suggests that we eat more beets, radishes, fennel, fenugreek, leafy greens and small amounts of cinnamon to thin the bile and thus making our pathways and delivery of enzymes faster and more efficient.

Benefits of Increasing Enzymes

1. Increases rate of recovery after disease.
2. Help transform and store energy.
3. Activates hormones.
4. Helps their own production.
5. Anti-inflammatory.
6. Enhance immune system by helping to control its regulatory mechanisms.
7. Increased energy.
8. Enhanced quality of living.
9. Dr. Mercola suggests that enzymes can help with digestion and assimilation of gluten and ultimately help with something like Celiac Disease.[15]

Direct Alternatives to Supplemental Digestive Enzymes — Tips from Dr. John Douillard[16]

1. Eat more *raw beets* and *leafy greens*. Greens should make up 2/3 of your plate. The cellulose in greens will attach to the toxic bile and escort it to the toilet like a non-stop flight!
2. *Drink fenugreek tea*. It acts as a decongestant for the bile ducts and helps support normal bile flow.
3. Have *cinnamon* with every meal. Cinnamon supports healthy blood sugar levels while supporting normal bile flow.
4. Mix 1-2 tbsp of *olive oil* with 1-2 tsp of *lemon juice*. Shake and drink every morning OR night on an empty stomach for 1 month. This will exercise the liver and gallbladder, while supporting healthy bile flow in the bile and pancreatic ducts.

---

15 http://articles.mercola.com/sites/articles/archive////gluten-part-three.asps
http://www.lifespan.com

16 https://lifespa.com/digestive-enzymes-the-hidden-dangers/

5. Drink a ***big glass of water*** 15-20 minutes before each meal. This will super-hydrate your stomach, encouraging it to produce more hydrochloric acid and increasing the flow of bile and pancreatic enzymes.

6. Consider ***regular detoxification*** of the liver and fat cells, which store toxins that are processed through the liver. Regular cleansing can help one achieve optimal digestion.

Protein
Where do you get your protein?

When I began to cut down on animal sourced protein, many people would ask the question: where do you get your protein? I thought to myself, "Why protein and not some other source of nutrition like fats or carbohydrates?" They were concerned about my health which was quite endearing; and at the time I did not have an answer. I relied on the wisdom of ancient traditions, like the Indian, where most of their culture is vegetarian and they didn't seem to be nutrient deficient. I had also met many vegans and vegetarians and they seemed to all be in good health.

In fact, the American Dietetic Association states that pure vegetarian diets contain about twice the daily need for protein. Harvard researchers suggest that it is difficult for vegetarians to become protein deficient unless they eat too much junk food or sweets.[17]

But still, where did I get my protein? Let's investigate protein.

What Is Protein?

Proteins are part of every cell, tissue and organ in the body — they are the building blocks of life. They are constantly being broken and down replaced (remember enzymes). Proteins are made up of amino acids. There are 21 different types of amino acids, 9 of which are considered to be essential amino acids. According to the Center for Disease Control the essential amino acids are those that cannot be made by humans.

17 *Conscious Eating,* Cousens p 312

When you see the term "complete protein," it means that the item is carrying all the essential amino acids.

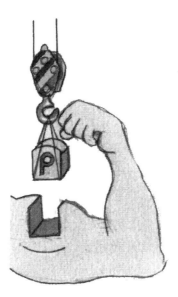

The body uses protein to make hormones and enzymes. Just like enzymes, proteins are used in numerous functions of the body from supporting the digestive and immune system, to boosting metabolism and muscle growth. Protein is an essential part for our overall health.

How Much Do I Need?

There are numerous opinions on how much protein you might need each day. According to many researchers and popular views, approximately 45 grams for women and 55 grams for men is the suggested daily intake. More and more science is showing us that 20-35 grams of protein is sufficient for men and women[18]. So who is really to say? My suggestion is that you are! These numbers are useful guidelines but you must use your own experience to really zero in on how much you need.

It's not as simple as grams though, because not all protein is created equal. The body will derive more usable protein from live plants than it will from cooked meats. The Max Planck Institute in Germany shows

---

18 *Conscious Eating,* Cousens p 312

that when you cook your protein you lose 50% of it in its actual form, i.e. 40 grams cooked = 20 grams live.[19]

Protein consumption and absorption depends on several factors: 1) how much you are moving; 2) how old you are; 3) the sources of protein; 4) your metabolic/dietary constitution.

Concerns About Over Consumption and Animal Sourced Protein

Overconsumption of protein can cause kidney issues, high blood pressure and heart issues. According to the Center for Disease Control, most Americans are eating too much protein.[20] "An excess-protein diet has been shown by the US Army to cause a deficiency of B6 and B3. Protein has also been found to leach out calcium, iron, zinc and magnesium from the system."[21] When our body becomes burdened with heavy, dense animal proteins it results in long term degeneration of our organism.

Osteoporosis is one example of this. The *Journal of Clinical Nutrition* in 1983 reported that: 1) female nonvegetarians had an average measurable bone loss of 35% compared with 7% bone loss in female vegetarians. 2) Male nonvegetarians had 18% bone loss compared with 3% vegetarians. "The evidence is overwhelming that the most important single dietary change one can make to prevent osteoporosis is to decrease the amount of protein in the diet."[22]

In general meats make the body acidic,[23] which, makes it more susceptible to diseases particularly osteoporosis and heart disease. Animal proteins, in general, are higher in saturated fats, which can elevate cholesterol levels and increase blood pressure.

Why does this happen? Well, animal proteins are not broken down easily, they can begin to putrefy becoming toxic — thus require more enzyme attention, immune support and they cause digestive disruption.

19 *Rainbow Green*, Cousens, p 56
20 http://www.cdc.gov/nutrition/everyone/basics/protein.html
21 *Conscious Eating*, Cousens p 314
22 *Conscious Eating*, Cousens p 315
23 *Conscious Eating*, Cousens p 177

The toxins (putrefied decaying fecal matter, especially related to these proteins) are pulled into the colon and can create strain on many organs. Our liver then needs to help by removing some of these stored toxins from our colon and intestines. Taxing our liver can create sludge and back up, therefore taxing the system even more (Remember Dr. Douillard and sludgy bile). The toxins that aren't removed are then pumped throughout the blood stream.

Sources for Protein

So, it is not essential that we all become vegetarians; but the data suggests that incorporating more plant based protein will not only give us more bio-available protein, it will also help prevent disease.

Good sources of complete veggie protein: almonds, sesame seeds, pumpkin seeds, sunflower seeds, soybeans, quinoa, buckwheat, peanuts, potatoes, all leafy greens and most fruits.

Other great sources of vegetarian protein are chlorella and spirulina. 3 tablespoons is a sufficient daily supply. 3 handfuls of nuts and seeds will also satisfy your protein cravings.

Benefits of Plant Based Protein

1) Decreased insulin resistance.
2) More bio-available.
3) Have alkalizing effects on the body
4) Get double amount of protein in the same amount of calories.
5) Lower in pathogenic microorganisms.
6) Add to our enzyme bank.
7) Lower risk of acidosis, osteoporosis, high cholesterol, heart disease, unhealthy bacterial growth in gut and premature aging.

Just E.A.T.

E = Enjoy **A** = Avoid **T** = Taste

When I first started exploring the notions of eating, I was excited about the possibilities. Reading and researching, I quickly became overwhelmed with the amount of information about food and nutrition. The different philosophies on diets and food scrambled my brain. The styles of cooking and food preparation were so vast I didn't know where to begin. The information on vitamins and supplements also became quite intimidating.

At some point in my research, I read that all these ideas about food and health were merely guidelines. They were all meant to be viewed through the lens of my personal experience. This lightened my mental load and the experiment began. I started trying different things and used my own inner wisdom to make proper choices for myself. I continued to find new, fresh tidbits of wisdom through my ongoing reading and research. These commonalties are shared below through the E.A.T. metaphor.

I encourage you to study, investigate, inquire, experiment and discover. Use your own intuition and guts to guide your choices. Be mindful that this could change over time and even day to day via new research and results. By using coming sense, honoring your body and adding valuable information, you can make the best food choices for yourself. Remember: there is no one diet for all people. We all have different preferences, body constitutions and moral commitments that we must factor into our food choices and preparation methods.

Enjoy

Enjoy these foods, beverages and ideas any day, any way.

1. Water

The basic structure of all life on earth is water — without water life does not exist. A crucial element in water is hydrogen for, "hydrogen molecule comprises 97% of the universe" (*Spiritual Nutrition* p. 475). Water's main function is to bring hydrogen to the body's cells so it becomes hydrated. It also eliminates toxins from cells by flushing them out. This is why it is beneficial to drink plenty of water when sick, not feeling 100% or after physical treatments or therapies of any kind.

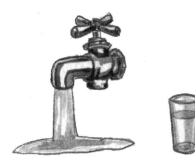

Our relationship with water is one of the most essential relationships we can cultivate. The average adult is 2/3 water or 50% of body weight (*Spiritual Nutrition* p. 480). It is important that we keep it that way. There are many symptoms of dehydration (they can also be called indicators to drink more). Some indicators include: dyspepsia, stomach pain; rheumatoid pain (arthritic pain) back pain can be due to discs not getting enough water; angina, heart pain; headaches; fatigue; restlessness (*Spiritual Nutrition* p. 482-483). Instead of going for a pill or searching for pharmaceutical remedies, try drinking water first. 75% of Americans are chronically dehydrated (*Spiritual Nutrition* p. 483). Many mistake thirst for hunger or the onset of a variety of physical ailments.

Drink, drink, and drink water. A good practice to get into is drinking 1 liter of water every morning upon waking. It helps get the metabolism going, flushes any toxins left from sleeping, cleanses the kidneys and provides the essential hydrogen your body craves. Try this instead of coffee or tea for one week and see how you feel.

Hydration Techniques

1. Drink 1 liter of water upon rising. This recommendation comes from many of my teachers and is offered by the film *Food Matters*.
2. Get a water bottle with measurements so you know how much you are drinking. Aim to consume 2-4 liters per day depending on how much you weigh and how much you exercise. Add lemon, cucumber or garden herbs for flavor.
3. Eat raw fruits and vegetables. They have high amounts of structured water and will help keep you hydrated.

4. Make 4 oz of saline solution by boiling water and adding sea salt until you can see the crystals in the water. This means it is saturated. Add 1/2 teaspoon for 1 liter of water.

5. Drink water in between meals. This will help with hunger cravings and keep you hydrated.

2. Organic Whole Food

What is organic food and how is it produced?

Organic farming is designed to encourage soil and water conservation and is aimed at reducing pollution. It also involves natural processes for managing crops by not using chemical pesticides and fertilizers. The following chart[24] clearly depicts the differences between conventional and organic farming.

CONVENTIONAL	ORGANIC
Apply chemical fertilizers to promote plant growth.	Apply natural fertilizers, such as manure or compost, to feed soil and plants.
Spray synthetic insecticides to reduce pests and disease.	Spray pesticides from natural sources; use beneficial insects and birds, mating disruption or traps to reduce pests and disease.
Use synthetic herbicides to manage weeds.	Use environmentally-generated plant-killing compounds; rotate crops, till, hand weed or mulch to manage weeds.
Give animals antibiotics, growth hormones and medications to prevent disease and spur growth.	Give animals organic feed and allow them access to the outdoors. Use preventive measures — such as rotational grazing, a balanced diet and clean housing — to help minimize disease.

24 akashafoodco.com

So now that we know a bit about organic farms and the methodology behind them, why is it important to grow and consume organic foods? What are the benefits of organic food and what are the risks of conventionally grown food?

Benefits of Organic Food

A study published by The Organic Center reveals that organic food is higher in certain key nutritional areas such as total antioxidant capacity, total polyphenols and two key flavonoids, quercetin and kaempferol, all of which are nutritionally significant.[25] A 2012 study in the *Journal of the Science of Food and Agriculture* discovered higher antioxidants, including vitamin C, in organic broccoli compared to conventional.[26]

Dr. Andrew Weil suggests we use organic food when pursuing optimum health. He points to a study presented by UC Davis in which they found that organic food has higher levels of cancer fighting agents than conventional food. The benefits of organic food are numerous, below is a list of just a few:

1. Higher antioxidants.
2. Less exposure to pesticides.
3. Less exposure to antibiotics and hormones. (Antibiotics lower intestinal flora in the gut.)
4. Less pollution, i.e. use of petrol chemicals, contamination of water supply and destabilization of soil.
5. They taste better.
6. Less risk of degenerative diseases.
7. They boost our digestive and immune systems.

Cost

Many of us are concerned about the price of organic food, and rightfully so. Sometimes when going to Whole Foods "like" grocery stores to get our organics we do spend more to eat clean and well. It is important

25   http://behindthescenes.org/organific/health/index.Phip
26   http://heartbreaking.Seagate.com/human-health-benefits-eating-organic-foods-.html

to place a higher value on our health and consider the hidden costs of the industrial production of food.

The cost of conventionally grown food is greater than we might think. Many of the processes and ingredients are subsidized by the government, so we are paying for them anyway. Much of the run-off from conventional farms renders the water undrinkable and the soil infertile. There is a greater risk for developing illness from pesticides, which in turn drives up the cost of healthcare.

According to *Omnivore's Dilemma*, by Michael Pollan, Americans spend less on food than any other industrialized country in the world. Is it really an affordability issue, or is it a matter of priority? When we begin to prioritize our health and our environment, we will see that eating organic food and supporting our local organic farmers is the better choice for our health.

Organic food is the largest growing sector of the food industry today. This is great news. The more we buy, the more farmers will be encouraged to produce organic food, which will, in turn, drive down the cost at the check out counter. Make organic food a priority and notice the health effects. Together we can make this a cost effective reality. It is time to reclaim our natural environment and the first step is buying organic.

3. Local and Seasonal

Local and seasonal (and organic) is one of the best ways to diversify your diet and provide your body with the highest amount of nutrition. Farmers markets and Community Supported Agriculture (CSAs) offer fresh foods that are picked at the height of their growing cycle ensuring the best nutrition. As the growing season progresses you will get a variety of foods based on your local climate – this is the way nature intended it. The CSAs may offer things that you are not used to buying. This is an opportunity to get creative with recipes and make something new.

By buying local, you also decrease carbon footprint and are able to build a relationship with the grower of your food. Shaking the hand that feeds you could be one of the most important things you can do for your health and happiness. Let food be thy medicine and your local farmer be your provider.

4. Fruits and Vegetables

Fruits and vegetables support a balanced acid/alkaline diet. They are high in vitamins, minerals and enzymes that help support circulation, blood purification, bone growth and they strengthen the immune system.

According to Richard DuBois, MD, Chief of Internal Medicine at Atlanta Medical Center and top authority on infectious disease, over 4500 studies show that whole fruits and veggies specifically prevent cancer. Andrew Weil, MD, probably the most famous Harvard-trained physician practicing alternative medicine in the world, recently stated: "A diet high in fruits and vegetables is associated with a lower risk of 15 types of cancer, among them, colon, breast, cervix and lung" (Silberstein 23).

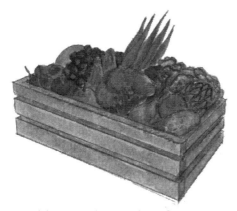

Fruits and vegetables get their colors from carotenoids, a large group of approximately 600 natural plant chemicals. Carotenes play two enormous roles in our health: 1) boost immune function 2) they are powerful antioxidants. Strong guts stimulate a healthy immune system and antioxidants help to destroy free radicals (free radicals are diseased cells that cause damage to the body).

Fruits and vegetables are rich in fiber. "The more fiber we consume, the more frequent and bulky are our solid eliminations through the bowels" (Silberstein p. 26). Fiber binds to toxic chemicals and helps to eliminate them through the bowels.

Vegetables, especially raw, are also a great source of protein. In fact, the American Dietetic Association states that pure vegetarian diets contain about twice the daily need for protein. Harvard researchers suggest that it is difficult for vegetarians to become protein deficient unless they eat too much junk food or sweets.[27]

How Much To Eat?

Susan Silberstein Ph.D., author of *Hungry for Health*, recommends that we eat "ideally 3 servings of fruit and 6-7 of veggies" (Silberstein p. 24). Remember the 80/20 rule from the acid/alkaline discussion. Cultures that eat 1 pound of fruits and vegetables per day have 50% less chance of getting western diseases. Vegetarians live longer and healthier lives than non-vegetarians (*In Defense of Food* p. 164).

Dark leafy greens are the best. "Green is my favorite color," my niece told me — a recent shift from pink. Of course, she was referring to the nutritive power of plants. Plants get their green color from chlorophyll, which is great for the blood. Its chemical make up is exactly the same as blood hemoglobin with the exception that the iron (in blood) is replaced by magnesium (plants). Plants are higher in bio-available calcium than dairy products. Eat as many dark leafy greens a day as possible.

5. Whole Grains

Whole grains can reduce the chance of heart disease, cancer and diabetes (*In Defense of Food* p. 110). Whole grains have all their fiber in tact, which helps to slow the grain from turning into sugar. They are a rich source of folic acid, antioxidants, fiber, vitamins and minerals. In 2003, the *American Journal of Clinical Nutrition* published a study demonstrating that subjects getting the same amounts of nutrients from different sources were not as healthy as whole grain eaters. This suggests the "whole" is greater than the sum of its parts.

---

27 *Conscious Eating*, Cousens p. 312

6. Home Cooked Meals

There is something about home cooking. Perhaps it's the smell from the kitchen. The care, attention and time taken to prepare can be an invigorating experience. There is a relationship that is established with our food when we take the time to cook it. We have a huge advantage when it comes to the ingredients we choose as well. Most likely you'll be using whole foods and spices that provide abundant amounts of nutrients. The likelihood of including high fructose corn syrup or partially hydrogenated oil in your food is greatly diminished — who even knows where to buy that stuff?

An added benefit is that it sparks creativity. We get a chance to learn, experiment and be alchemists during the cooking process. This feeds us in many other ways beside just our body. Lastly, by cooking our own food, the body has time to start its digestive process and prepare for the consumption and integration of nutrients.

7. Superfoods

Some health experts have begun classifying certain "superfoods" in their own category. They are certain types of food that are supercharged with beneficial nutrition. These truly are foods that heal. Superfoods are an essential component for experiencing Robust Vitality. They are the best medicines on the planet – incorporate them into your nutritional lifestyle! Superfoods are easily added to your diet. See Section 11 for a full description of recommended superfoods and their uses.

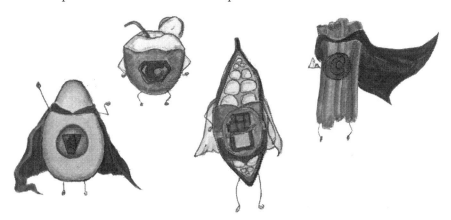

8. Juice

Fresh vegetable and fruit juice (NOT pre-made, store bought juice) is a great addition to any diet. They are loaded with vitamins, minerals and enzymes that your body has easy access to. Raw juice (80% vegetable) is anti-inflammatory, alkalizing and highly nutritious.

By juicing your fruits and vegetables, most of the fiber is removed, leaving the vital nutrients in an easily digestible form. Because juice only has trace amounts of fiber it is able to enter the blood stream faster than whole foods. This is not only highly alkalizing, but allows your digestion to relax so your body can use its energy for detoxification and cellular repair. Your body uses the benefits of juice as medicine by cleaning, restoring and revitalizing your cells (Dr. Max Gerson's work). It is as if you are taking vitamin pills in liquid form.

Fresh juice is gaining popularity in the West. There are juice shops in every major city. The movie *Fat, Sick and Nearly Dead*, created by Joe Cross, has inspired hundreds of thousands of people to start juicing. He was severely overweight, had an autoimmune disease and was taking multiple medications. After a 60-day juice fast (which he documented in his film), he lost over 80 pounds, cured himself of his auto-immune disease and kicked all of his medication. He is now one of the leading advocates for juicing. I have had the pleasure of working with him managing the juice production for several hundred people as they juice cleanse. It is amazing to see so many people coming to this practice to heal their bodies.

A good balance for juice is along the same lines as the 80/20 rule: 80% vegetables and 20% fruit.

9. Smoothies

Smoothies are a great way to get vital nutrients into the body in effective and delicious ways. Smoothies are blended fruits and vegetables that are easily digestible. Since the liquefying process breaks down the cell walls in food, our body can assimilate their nutritional essence easier than whole foods. They are also an easy way to incorporate more fruits, vegetables and superfoods into your diet. Get creative and enjoy a delicious smoothie. Do your best to include as many vegetables as possible.

Benefits

1. They are quick and easy meals to make that are delicious and portable.
2. They help improve digestion because they are not as much of a burden on your digestive system. The blender has already pre-chewed your food.
3. They are an easy way to get your daily-recommended fruits and vegetables.
4. They tend to be lower in calories because they contain high amounts of water and fiber.
5. They help with losing weight because they help fight hunger and cravings by making you feel full and provide your necessary vitamins and minerals.
6. They help you stay hydrated.

Avoid

Avoid everyday, every way.

1. Pesticides

Pesticides were developed post WWII as a byproduct from the old military industrial complex. Left over materials were converted into DDT (which is now banned) and a variety of other pesticides. They were then (and are still) used on crops to attempt to control insects and pests from damaging our food. We now know that many of these pesticides are quite harmful to our health and environment.

Pesticides disrupt the endocrine system, the system that regulates our hormones, which in turn effects our organs and every cell in our body. Upsetting the balance of our hormones can lead to infertility and

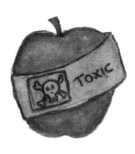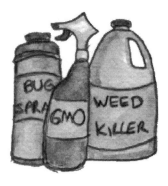

a variety of birth defects.[28] The US Environmental Protection Agency, considers 60% of herbicides, 90% of fungicides and 30% of insecticides as potentially cancer causing.[29]

Pesticides are stored in the colon where they, over time, poison the body. Your colon is the last organ in your digestive system. Some Eastern cultures base the health of their elderly on the strength of their colon. We are seeing colon cancer and digestive problems on the rise in the US, could this be part of the reason?[30]

Countless studies have linked pesticide contamination with cancer, Alzheimer's disease, Parkinson's disease,[31] ADHD, infertility, muscular diseases, etc.[32]

Pesticides Impact On Our Children

Children have a higher health risk when coming into contact with chemicals because of the underdevel- opment of their immune system.

28   http://fooddemocracy.wordpress.com/2008/01/18/the-dirty-dozen-12-foodsfood-additives-to-avoid-and-why/ Please visit this website for more information on foods and chemicals to avoid. Not listed in the "avoid" section are: BHA and BHT, Sodium Nitrate and Nitrite, and Brominated Vegetable Oil (BVO). Please note than any footnote referenced as www.fooddemocracy.com is excerpted from a post in the January 2008 issue by Kelly Scotti, and supplemented with information by the Center for Science in the Public Interest http://www.cspinet.org/reports/chemcuisine.html

29   http://www.toxicsaction.org/problems-and-solutions/pesticides

30   http://www.care2.com/greenliving/17-essential-reasons-to-eat-organic-food.html

31   http://beyondpesticides.org/organicfood/health/index.php

32   Research from Harvard University School of Public Health found that 70% increase in Parkinson's in people exposed to pesticides. http://www.care2.com/greenliving/17-essential-reasons-to-eat-organic-food.html

Their brains and organs have not fully matured and therefore cannot process toxicity the way adults do. A study from the University of Montreal and Harvard University, May 2010, suggested that pesticides may double the risk for children developing ADHD.[33] In February 2009, The Agency for Toxic Substances and Disease Registry published a study that in homes where pesticides were used, children were twice as likely to develop brain cancer versus those that did not.[34]

Cancer and ADHD are a few of the more publicized health risks associated with childhood toxicity from pesticides, but studies are showing that everything from allergies, digestive issues, energy levels and even anxiety can be a result of a stressed immune system.

The Dirty Dozen

The Dirty Dozen[35] is a list of the most pesticide toxic fruits and vegetables on the market. Avoid buying them if they are not organic. The Clean Fifteen are also listed below. These are the fruits and vegetables that are the most resistant to pesticides and less toxic if grown conventionally.

DIRTY DOZEN:

1) Apples 2) Strawberries 3) Grapes 4) Celery 5) Peaches 6) Spinach 7) Sweet bell peppers 8) Nectarines (imported) 9) Cucumbers 10) Cherry tomatoes 11) Snap peas (imported) 12) Potatoes

THE CLEAN FIFTEEN:

1) Avocados 2) Sweet corn 3) Pineapples 4) Cabbage 5) Sweet peas (frozen) 6) Onions 7) Asparagus 8) Mangos 9) Papayas 10) Kiwi 11) Eggplant 12) Grapefruit 13) Cantaloupe 14) Cauliflower 15) Sweet potatoes

---

33 http://beyondpesticides.org/organicfood/health/index.php

34 http://www.toxicsaction.org/problems-and-solutions/pesticides

35 http://www.mindbodygreen.com/0-13571/12-fruits-veggies-with-the-most-pesticides-2014-dirty-dozen.html This List comes from many other sources as well including Dr. Weil's work.

2. Genetically Modified Foods

Genetically Modified Organisms (GMOs) are plants and animals that have been engineered, altered and changed to withstand pesticides and/or produce their own insecticides.[36] In the US, the majority of the corn, soybean, cotton and canola crops are now genetically modified. GMOs are used in about 80% of all processed foods.[37] Questions about their safety arise with regularity — in fact, they have never been proven to be safe.[38] The companies that make them advertise that they are safe, but more and more research strongly suggests the opposite.

In fact, more than 60 countries around the world, including Australia, Japan and all the countries in the European Union have significant restrictions or outright bans on these products.[39] Do they know something that we don't?

GMOs are also a detriment to our environment. They have caused a rise in the use of pesticides and an emergence of what are being called "superweeds" and "superbugs."[40] These "superpests" are detrimental to our health and our environment. They cause crop damage, soil pollution and water spoilage. Irradiation, antibiotics, and more pesticides are then used to control these outbreaks further increasing the risk to our health and environment.

It is best practice to avoid GMOs altogether.

---

36 18% of all GMO are designed to produce their own pesticides. Research is showing that these crops still grow pesticides inside your body. http://www.care2.com/greenliving/17-essential-reasons-to-eat-organic-food.html

37 http://www.nongmoproject.org/learn-more/

38 www.fooddemocracy.com: GMOs have not been proven to be safe and some studies show GMO's may decrease immunity to diseases in plants as well as humans, may cause resistance to antibiotics and may have a negative impact on genetic function.

39 http://www.nongmoproject.org/learn-more/

40 www.fooddemocracy.com

3. Artificial Sweeteners and Colors/High Fructose Corn Syrup

Artificial sweeteners are a combination of chemicals that exist to make our foods sweeter without the calories of sugar. Most artificial sweeteners have side effects, and their chemical breakdown in the body can be toxic. In addition, in combination with other food additives like artificial colors and sweeteners can have a much more potent effect on nerve cells. Artificial sweeteners have been linked to over 90 side effects.[41]

Artificial colors are synthetic chemicals that do not occur in nature. Most are derived from coal tar and can contain up to 10 parts per million of lead and arsenic and still be recognized as safe by the FDA. Artificial colors can cause allergic reaction, hyperactivity, ADHD in children, and may contribute to visual and learning disorders, and cause nerve damage.

High fructose corn syrup is a highly processed derivative of corn. It is a relatively new addition to the human diet and has proven to be a detriment to the body's health. It can only be processed in the liver, which is not ideal because it must produce higher levels of cholesterol to absorb it. High fructose corn syrup affects the way your brain recognizes and therefore regulates food consumption. High fructose corn syrup resists leptin absorption in the brain, which is the protein that is vital for regulating energy intake and expenditure.

Processed sugars, high fructose corn syrup, and artificial sweeteners are to be avoided. Therefore sodas, cookies, sweets and anything with processed sugar are a huge detriment to the body and a major factor in contributing to heart disease, diabetes and obesity.

4. Ingredients You Cannot Pronounce or Recognize as Food

If you need a chemical engineering degree to figure out what the ingredient is in your food, then you either go back to school or don't eat

---

41 www.fooddemocracy.com

it. If you can't recognize the name or pronounce it, then re-study phonics or don't eat it. In the book, *In Defense of Food*, Michael Pollan suggests that we don't eat anything that our grandmother wouldn't recognize as food (p.148). This is a great guideline for simplifying our food choices. Read the labels on your food to test your scientific skills.

5. Soda

Most soda is highly toxic because of the artificial colors, sweeteners and high sugar content. Many believe that soda should come with a warning label just like cigarettes – Danger: May lead to obesity, diabetes, osteoporosis and heart issues. Diet, caffeine free and regular soda are all known culprits in the obesity epidemic.

Hazards of Soda

1. Soda has approximately 10 teaspoons of sugar, which will spike blood sugar and can result in insulin resistance, diabetes, and obesity.
2. Most soda has caffeine (see risks of caffeine in the Taste section).
3. Soda contains phosphoric acid, which interferes with the body's ability to absorb calcium. It also slows digestion and blocks nutrient absorption.
4. The water used to make soda is tap water, which can contain chlorine, fluoride and heavy metals.
5. Soda causes dehydration.
6. Soda causes plaque to build up in your teeth which can stain your teeth, cause gum disease and tooth decay.
7. Hannah Gardner, Ph.D. at the University of Miami led a study that showed daily diet soda drinkers have a 48% higher chance of heart attack and stroke than nondaily soda drinkers.[42]

---

42 http://www.webmd.com/diet/features/sodas-and-your-health-risks-debated

Risks of Soda

Soda stimulates the dopamine productive in the brain, giving you a high similar to a drug addict..

Most soda has caffeine (see risks of caffeine in the Taste section), such as acidifying the body, causing emotional imbalance and dehydration.

Soda causes plaque to build up in your teeth which can stain your teeth, cause gum disease and tooth decay.

The water used to make soda is tap water, which can contain chlorine, fluoride and heavy metals. ⊠ They all are toxin to a certain degree which can effect the liver,brain and immune system.

Hannah Gardner, Ph.D. at the University of Miami led a study that showed daily diet soda drinkers have a 48% higher chance of heart attack and stroke than nondailysoda drinkers. 1

Many soft drink cans and plastic bottles contain Bisphenyl-A (BPA). Because of its toxic effects on the endocrine system, BPAhas been linked to caner, premature puberty and reproductive issues.

The phosphoric acid in sodas has been linked to kidney stones.The caffeine taxes your adrenals and kidneys, effecting your energy levels, mood and causes dehydration.

Soda has approximately 10 teaspoons of sugar, which will spike blood sugar and can result in insulin resistance, diabetes, and obesity.

Soda contains phosphoric acid, which interferes with the body's ability to absorb calcium. It also slows digestion and blocks nutrient absorption. This can lead to osteoporosis.

6. Hydrogenated and Partially Hydrogenated Oils

Partially hydrogenated vegetable oil is made by reacting vegetable oil with hydrogen. When this hydrogenation process occurs, a healthful fatty acid (polyunsaturated) is converted into a harmful one (trans). They contribute to high cholesterol levels because they actually scar the interior walls of your arteries. This continual scarring slowly shrinks the opening for blood to flow through. The blood also thickens and has a harder time pumping through the arteries and to the body's organs. This places undue strain on the heart and slows brain function. Decreased blood circulation can lead to various emotional and physical ailments such an Alzheimer's, Parkinson's, ADHD and mental confusion just to name a few.[43]

The Natural News online publication re-affirms these dangers with and excerpt from *The Guide to Healthy Eating* by M.D. David Brownstein.[44]

> *The downside for consumers is the dangerous trans fats that are formed with hydrogenation. The ingestion of partially hydrogenated vegetable oils and the trans fats that are formed with this process has been linked to increases in cancer, heart disease, and many other chronic degenerative disorders. What is wrong with trans fats? Trans fats, formed during hydrogenation, are actually toxic substances for our cell membranes. When our cells contain an overabundance of trans fats, the cells become leaky and distorted. This can promote vitamin and mineral deficiencies.*

Partially hydrogenated oils can be found in many snack foods, cookies, pastries, margarines, and deep-fried foods. Read food labels and only purchase products with 0 trans fats.

---

43 http://www.greenpasture.org/fermented-cod-liver-oil-butter-oil-vitamin-d-vitamin-a/why-hydrogenated-oils-should-be-avoided-at-all-costs-submitted-by-dr-donald/

44 http://www.naturalnews.com/027445_fat_fats_trans.html

7. Monosodium Glutamate (MSG)

Monosodium Glutamate (MSG), a salt that is chemically converted to bring out the flavor in foods, is one of the worst food additives on the market. MSG is an excitotoxin. According to Dr. Russell Blaylock, author of *Excitotoxins: The Taste that Kills* and practicing neurosurgeon, excitotoxins can cause sensitive neurons to die. This means that MSG overexcites your brain cells to the point of damage, acting as a poison.

Excitotoxins are amino acids that function as neurotransmitters. They over stimulate the brain, damage the hypothalamus (area of brain that regulates hunger) and cause the release of excess dopamine giving the body the junky like rush. Essentially it damages the hardwiring of the brain, which is not only linked cravings, but a whole host of other issues such as headaches, itchy skin, dizziness, respiratory, digestive, and circulatory issues.[45] It is also most certainly linked to obesity,[46] type 2 diabetes and liver damage.

Here are some of the code names used for these additives: hydrolyzed protein, hydrolyzed plant protein, plant protein extract, sodium caseinate, calcium caseinate, yeast extract, textured protein, autolyzed yeast, hydrolyzed oat flour. These additives ALWAYS contain MSG. Be on the lookout for the following additives as well because they also indicate MSG and/or other excitotoxins: malt extract, malt flavoring, bouillon, broth, stock, flavoring, natural flavoring, natural beef or chicken flavoring, seasoning, spices, carrageenan, enzymes, soy protein concentrate, soy protein isolate, whey protein concentrate.[47]

8. The Microwave

Just the concept of "nuking" something, especially your food, should make you suspicious. So what is microwaving exactly and why do we

---

45 www.fooddemocracy.com

46 http://articles.mercola.com/sites/articles/archive/2007/08/28/dangers-of-msg.aspx

47 http://foodmatters.tv/articles-1/the-dangers-of-msg

call it nuking? Microwaves heat food by causing water molecules in it to resonate at very high frequencies and eventually turn to steam, which heats your food.[48] This process heats your food rapidly from the inside out and causes a change in your food's chemical structure. Microwaving food is a form of irradiation, hence the term "nuking."

According to Mike Adams, the Health Ranger and editor of NaturalNews.com,

*Microwaved food is not merely "dead" food at every level, it is food that has been **molecularly deconstructed,** leaving nothing but empty calories, fiber and minerals. Virtually the entire vitamin and phytonutrient content has been destroyed.*[49]

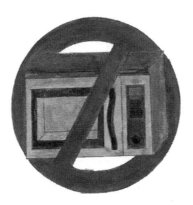

Destruction of food and its essential nutrients is not the only hazard to using a microwave. The January/February issue of *Nutrition Action Newsletter*[50] reported the leakage of toxic chemicals from microwavable food packaging. Some of these chemicals included polyethylene terpthalate (PET), benzene, toluene, and xylene – say what? By microwaving, especially fatty foods, carcinogens and other toxic chemicals are released.

9. Sugar

Sugar is used to supply energy to the body. It helps with many of the body's systems such as stimulating the pancreas to produce insulin

48   http://articles.mercola.com/sites/articles/archive/2010/05/18/microwave-hazards.aspx
49   http://www.naturalnews.com/039404_microwave_ovens_vitamins_nutrients.html#
50   http://articles.mercola.com/sites/articles/archive/2010/05/18/microwave-hazards.aspx

to balance the blood sugar. There are two main types of sugar: glucose and fructose. Glucose is primary energy source for our brains, cellular functions such as transportation and production of the bodies essential biological chemicals. Your brain receives information from glucose that it has had enough to eat and will stop consuming food. The body uses glucose in other beneficial ways such as regulating energy consumption, transferring nutrients throughout the body and aiding in elimination.

Fructose, on the other hand, can only be processed in the liver, which is not ideal because it must produce higher levels of cholesterol to absorb it. Fructose affects the way your brain recognizes and therefore regulates consumption. Fructose, unlike glucose, resists the leptin, which is the protein vital for regulating energy intake and expenditure. Processed sugars, high fructose corn syrup, and artificial sweeteners are to be avoided. Therefore sodas, cookies, sweets and anything with processed sugar are a huge detriment to the body and a major factor in contributing to heart disease, diabetes and obesity. Fruit juices and dried fruits can also have the same deleterious affects as refined sugars, are thus also addictive and should be consumed in moderation.

Hazards of Sugar

1. Sugar is highly addictive.[51]

Researchers at Princeton University studying animals binging on sugar, suggest that their brain behavior mimics that of people who abuse drugs like heroin and cocaine. "Our evidence from an animal model suggests that bingeing on sugar can act in the brain in ways very similar to drugs of abuse," says lead researcher and Princeton psychology professor Bart Hoebel.[52]

Dr. Robert Lustig, Professor of Pediatrics in the Division of Endocrinology at the University of California has explained the addictive nature of sugar as follows:

---

51 An informative article about sugar and addiction: http://www.bloomberg.com/news/2011-11-02/fatty-foods-addictive-as-cocaine-in-growing-body-of-science.html

52 http://www.nydailynews.com/life-style/health/sugar-addictive-cocaine-heroin-studies-suggest-article-1.356819

"The brain's pleasure center, called the nucleus accumbens, is essential for our survival as a species... Turn off pleasure, and you turn off the will to live... But long-term stimulation of the pleasure center drives the process of addiction... When you consume any substance of abuse, including sugar, the nucleus accumbens receives a dopamine signal, from which you experience pleasure. And so you consume more.

The problem is that with prolonged exposure, the signal attenuates, gets weaker. So you have to consume more to get the same effect—tolerance. And if you pull back on the substance, you go into withdrawal. Tolerance and withdrawal constitute addiction. And make no mistake, sugar is addictive."[53]

2. Sugar can suppress the immune system. Limiting the body's natural defenses for warding off disease.

3. Sugar interferes with absorption of calcium and magnesium.

4. Sugar can cause a rapid rise of adrenaline levels in children.

5. Sugar can make our skin age by changing the structure of collagen.

6. Sugar can increase the body's fluid retention.

7. High consumption of sugar and the corresponding elevated insulin levels can cause weight gain, bloating, fatigue, arthritis, headaches/migraines, weakened eyesight, lowered immune function, obesity, cavities, cardiovascular disease and increased cholesterol.

8. Sugar can also disrupt absorption of nutrients, possibly leading to cancer, Alzheimer's disease, osteoporosis, depression, PMS symptoms and stress.

9. Sugar can disrupt sleeping patterns especially if eaten later in the day.

10. Technology

When eating, it is best to avoid technological devices like televisions, computers and smartphones. When we are not aware and present with

---

53 http://articles.mercola.com/sites/articles/archive/2013/07/18/brain-imaging-confirms-food-addiction.aspx

our food, our bodies do not digest well. Mechanical impulses kick-in and overeating is likely. The brains is focused on something other than consuming food; therefore, it does not know when to tell us to stop eating. Eating in front of a computer could be worse than being in front of a television. Not only is the bacteria at your workstation much higher than that on a kitchen table; but, the electromagnetic fields from the computer poison your food and water (similar to what happens in a microwave).

Taste

Taste just a little bit, once in while.

1. Dairy

The consumption of milk (and dairy products in general like cheese and butter) after infancy is unnatural and unhealthy. Most humans between 18 months and age 4 lose the enzyme lactase, which is necessary to digest dairy.[54] This is why so many people in our culture are lactose intolerant.

Despite what the meat and dairy industry would say, dairy is not a good source of protein or calcium. In fact, it leaches calcium from the bones (can you say osteoporosis?). Most dairy cows are treated with hormones and antibiotics in order for them to survive their penned, grain feed, motionless lifestyles. In India, cows are considered sacred — this is a stark difference to the way cows are treated in the US.

Indians use what is called ghee or clarified butter as a fat/protein source for delivering nutrients to the body. Use ghee instead of butter.

The process of pasteurization does not effectively kill all bacteria and viruses and in turn destroys the live enzymes we would need to digest it. If you are going to eat dairy products, do so in moderation. Yogurt can be a useful source of probiotic enzymes, but make sure it is cultured. Greek yogurt and kefir are sources for these live probiotics.

---

54 *Conscious Eating* p. 479

Dr. Gabriel Cousens sums up dairy consumption best:

The answer to the dairy question is that if one does not have milk intolerance, does not easily produce mucus, does not mind being exposed to increased concentrations of toxins, bacteria, and radioactive substances, does not have a milk allergy, does not care about taking on a victim consciousness in every sip or clogging arteries and subtle energetic channels, does not mind increased weight gain, making your body more acidic, or contributing to the destruction of ecology, then dairy is acceptable in moderation (Conscious Eating 481).

Think of dairy as a condiment, delicacy or a treat for special occasions. It should not be a major part of your dietary intake.

2. Restaurant Food

I've worked in the food service industry for over 15 years and have seen what comes in and out of a kitchen. Most of the food you are being served comes from mass-market distributors and is not close to quality food. It has been produced, packaged and shipped in ways that are toxic to your health and destructive for the environment.

Not only are the ingredients potentially hazardous to your health, but also the preparation is based around speed and flavor — most restaurants do not have your health in mind. They use lots of low quality fats to enhance flavoring. Many of the cooking methods are designed to yield high amounts. Cleanliness and care are lower on the list of importance as well.

If you are going out to eat, one of my favorite things to do is look at the cleanliness of the ceilings and the top shelves. If the ceiling is clean you know that the restaurant is paying attention to cleanliness in other places.

When you go out to eat, go out to eat. It is your time to splurge. It is your time to have that dessert, to forget about all the rules and just enjoy! Never ever feel guilty. If you feel guilty, you're impacting your dining experience and actually ingesting that emotion. If you are going to have something that you "know" is not healthy, love it just the way you would anything else.

Still, avoid letting fast food options become anything close to regular.

3. Animal Protein

In general meats make the body acidic,[55] which, makes you more susceptible to diseases particularly osteoporosis and heart disease. Animal proteins are not broken down easily, they can begin to putrefy becoming toxic — thus require more enzyme attention, immune support and cause digestive disruption. The toxins (putrefied decaying fecal matter, especially related to these proteins) are pulled into the colon and can create strain on our organs. Our liver then needs to help by removing some of these stored toxins from our colon and intestines. The toxins that aren't removed are then pumped throughout the blood stream. Taxing our liver can create sludge and back up, therefore taxing the entire system even more (Remember Dr. Douillard and sludgy bile).

According to the Center for Disease Control most Americans are eating too much protein.[56] "An excess-protein diet has been shown by the US Army to cause a deficiency of B6 and B3. Protein has also been found to leach out calcium, iron, zinc and magnesium from the system."[57] When our body becomes burdened with heavy, dense animal proteins it results in long term degeneration of our organism. Animal proteins, in general, are higher in saturated fats, which, can elevate our cholesterol levels and increase blood pressure. Overconsumption of protein can cause kidney issues, heart issues and colon distress.

Osteoporosis is another example of overconsumption. The *Journal of Clinical Nutrition* in 1983 reported that: 1) female non-vegetarians had an average measurable bone loss of 35% compared with 7% bone loss in female vegetarians. 2) Male non-vegetarians had 18% bone loss compared with 3% vegetarians. "The evidence is overwhelming that the most important single dietary change one can make to prevent osteoporosis is to decrease the amount of protein in the diet."[58]

---

55 *Conscious Eating*, Cousens p 177
56 http://www.cdc.gov/nutrition/everyone/basics/protein.html
57 *Conscious Eating*, Cousens p 314
58 *Conscious Eating*, Cousens p 315

Industrial animal husbandry in the US, for the most part, is unnatural and destructive. These animals are fed foods that they did not evolve to eat, are kept in quite horrific conditions and are pumped with hormones and antibiotics in order to prevent diseases (which are a result of their diet and lifestyle). Environmentally, the industrial meat industry is one of the worst when it comes to abusing natural resources and is a large polluter of land and water.

In general, we no longer need the animal protein the way we used to because of our sedentary lifestyle. Our body and teeth are also designed in a way that suggest we eat a mostly plant based diet anyway. Remember the 80/20 rule when eating meat and make meat the 20.

If you are going to consume meat, it is best to get a share in a locally raised and slaughtered animal. Then freeze it. Make sure it is pasteurized grass finished. Grass finished means it has had grass throughout its entire life. Thomas Jefferson suggested eating meat as a flavor principle or as a condiment for vegetables.

Check out www.eatwild.com for more information on meat.

4. Caffeine

Caffeine is a plant compound that is commonly found in coffee, tea, chocolate, snack foods and gum. It is a stimulant that has addictive qualities. Even though in small amounts it maybe ok, overconsumption is prevalent. In general, caffeine is not the best long-term health choice.

The Risks of Caffeine

1. Caffeine blocks iron absorption in guts and prevents the kidneys ability to retain calcium, zinc, magnesium and other minerals. It causes calcium to be excreted from the bones, which can lead to osteoporosis and increase infertility.
2. Caffeine is a diuretic, which easily leads to dehydration.
3. Coffee is acidic and causes an acidic environment in the body. It thins the stomach lining, again, not good for IBS, Crohn's, or ulcers.

4. Caffeine relaxes esophageal sphincter, which can contribute to acid reflux (hydrochloric acid launches back up esophagus and burns lining).

5. Caffeine stimulates peristalsis and gastric emptying which pushes food into small intestines before it is finished digesting.

6. Coffee is one of the most pesticide intensive crops in the world.

7. Acrylamide is a potential carcinogen. It is released from roasting beans. The darker the roast, the higher the acrylamide.

8. Coffee stains your teeth and affects the quality of your taste buds.

9. Caffeine increases heart rate, tension and stress levels in the body. Blocks Gamma-aminobutyric acid (GABA), which is a neuro-transmitter that regulates mood and stress.

10. Coffee stimulates hydrochloric acid in gut. We need hydrochloric acid to digest food especially protein. When undigested protein gets passed to the small intestines it can cause bloating, irritable bowel syndrome (IBS), constipation and a variety of other ailments. As we get older our ability to create hydrochloric acid diminishes. Studies show that at least 37% of people over the age of 60 are HCL deficient and as many as 98% of people are impaired.

Coffee can be tricky because there are some beneficial health results showing in statistics.[59] Many people that drink coffee abuse the benefits of it and use it as a crutch rather than a health benefit or detoxification tool. If you are stressed or in a state of "fight or flight" (sympathetic nervous system dominance), coffee is not recommended. If and when you drink coffee, have it slowly and drink it as a ritual, rather than out of habit.

Detoxifying from caffeine can often lead to headaches and achiness. This is ok; it is all part of the process. Your body might undergo some changes during caffeine detoxification and sometimes discomfort is part of the process. This is typically referred to as a healing crisis. I encourage you to push through and rest during these potential experiences.

---

59 *Brain Maker*, by David Perlmutter points to research showing the coffee can help to decrease the risk of Alzheimer's and certain types of cancer.

A cautionary note on de-caffeinated beverages: De-caffeinated beverages are highly processed and usually require chemicals to eliminate the caffeine. They are not healthy alternatives. Consider drinking beverages that are naturally free of caffeine.

5. Alcohol

According to *In Defense of Food*, by Michael Pollan those people that drink moderately and regularly live longer and have less chance of heart disease than those that don't (p. 181). It's very important to consider the pattern and timing of drinking alcohol. It is best consumed with food and having small amounts daily rather than binging on the weekends. This is the perfect example of the "everything in moderation" motto.

Even though alcohol can be detrimental to your health, it has a place in various rituals and celebrations. As there are problems with addiction in our society, please contemplate your consumption. I do not recommend getting intoxicated, nor do I suggest having more than a glass of wine with dinner.

6. The Things You Know are Unhealthy but Absolutely Love

Apply this rule to everything but the avoid section. This process is not about suffering as one of my teachers likes to say. It is about empowered awareness, encouragement, growth and *robust vitality*. There are going to be some things that give your spirit a lift, that remind you of your childhood or that just put a smile on your face. For me it has been Oreo cookies. I would allow myself to enjoy these treats even though I knew they were toxic. After working on my physical, mental and emotional development, I now no longer see these cookies as food. In fact, they look more like science experiments and cause upset in my stomach.

Techniques
The ABCs

Awareness: When eating, it is useful to take the approach that this is a total sensory experience. Notice everything: the table and how it is set, the people who will be enjoying the meal with you, and the overall feel of the room. When served, look at the food and observe what you will be eating: the colors, the different types of food and how it is presented on the plate. Is there steam coming from the dish? What colors do you see? What does it smell like? How is your posture? Take a moment to take it all in, do not rush. Take a few breaths and center before biting in.

Blessing: The food did not magically appear on the plate and you did not just materialize in front of it. Settle in and let go of everything that came before the meal. You are there to eat, so be present. Bring to mind the notion of gratitude and thanks: gratitude for the earth, the farmers, the deliverer of the produce, the chef and all the other factors that contributed to the food. Give thanks and praise for the food and your ability to enjoy in one of the most essential practices for sustaining and uplifting your existence. This is a time to invoke any spiritual practices you may follow. Aloud or to yourself, make a blessing then enjoy.

Chewing: One of the most important things that we can do to be conscious eaters is to chew, chew, chew. This might seem simple, but according to *The Trenton Times* Monday, September 22, 2013 approximately 4000 people die a year from choking (information comes from Center for Disease Control and Prevention). These numbers are inspiration enough to be more mindful about how we eat. We always teach our children to chew their food, so let us do it with great care as an example for our children.

Take a minute to think, smell and then chew. The more we chew the easier it is for our bodies to assimilate the nutrition offered by the food. Particularly denser foods like meat and fish, it is the utmost importance that we chew to the max.

Some techniques for mindful chewing:

1. Take small bites.
2. When you think you are done chewing, chew 20 more times.
3. Put your utensil down and sit back in between bites. Savor each bite, and then resume eating.
4. Use your nondominant hand when handling utensils.
5. Use your hands to eat. Many cultures embrace this eating practice. Try it; your kids will love it.

Slow: Eat slowly. Take time for your meals so you can enjoy them. By eating slowly we give our body time to process the food we are eating, which will make for greater assimilation of nutrients and less digestive issues. We can also more fully enjoy the company we are with. Celebrate eating at every meal, everyday.

The 80/20 Rule

The 80/20 rule is simple: During a meal eat 80% alkaline-forming foods, and 20% acid-forming foods. Not all acid-forming foods are bad. Some acid-forming foods are necessary for nutritional value and for proper pH balance.

In Okinawa, Japan they eat up to 80% full to give their body and brain time to integrate it's food experience. Some research suggests that it takes about 20 minutes for your brain to recognize the body is full. So, there it is again, the 80/20 rule.

Food Plate

What's on your food plate? The diagram next page shows a great guideline for designing your plate. Broad categories give you the ability to choose your own style within healthy parameters. This is enhanced from the USDA's version from choosemyplate.gov (now the current replacement for the "food pyramid").

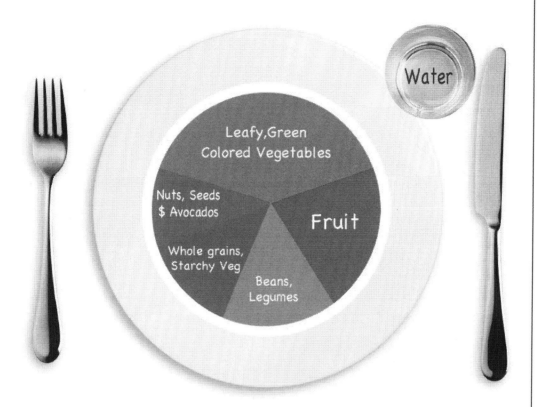

Food Combining[60]

One of the things that many nutritionists agree on is food combining. The body secretes different enzymes for different foods. Best practice is to consume foods that will help each other digest rather than compete in the stomach. Improper food combinations can cause stomach pain, heartburn, bloating, constipation and IBS. Some basics for food combining:

1. Eat fruits on their own and melons away from other fruits.
2. Proteins and starches do not mix well. Sorry, no more meat and potatoes.
3. Eat greens. Greens are great for digestion and combine well with almost all other foods.
4. Timing. Space out your meals and be mindful of these basic guidelines: wait two hours after eating fruit, three hours after eating starches and four hours after eating protein.

---

60 helpful resources for food combining: http://www.trueactivist.com/6-food-combining-rules-for-optimal-digestion/ http://mostlyraw.eu/2011/07/12/introduction-to-food-combining/

FOOD COMBINING CHART

- Eat Proteins and Carbohydrates at different meals
- Eat only one concentrated protein at each meal
- Treat juices (Fruit or Vegetable) as whole food

- Take milk alone or not at all
- Desert desserts
- Cold foods (including liquids) inhibit digestion

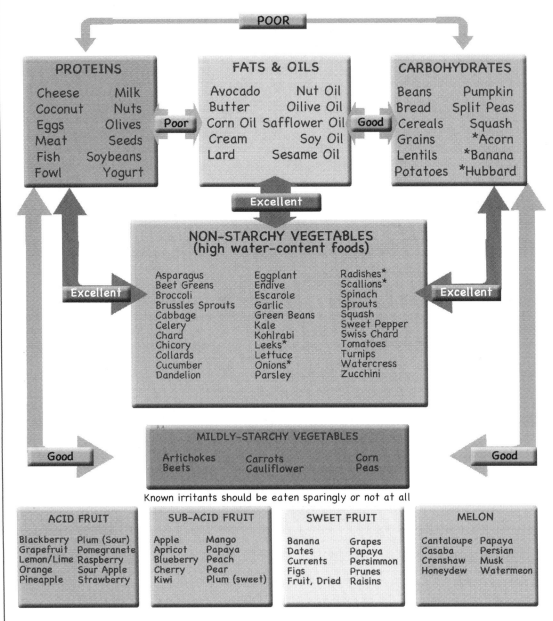

POOR

PROTEINS

Cheese	Milk
Coconut	Nuts
Eggs	Olives
Meat	Seeds
Fish	Soybeans
Fowl	Yogurt

FATS & OILS

Avocado	Nut Oil
Butter	Oilive Oil
Corn Oil	Safflower Oil
Cream	Soy Oil
Lard	Sesame Oil

CARBOHYDRATES

Beans	Pumpkin
Bread	Split Peas
Cereals	Squash
Grains	*Acorn
Lentils	*Banana
Potatoes	*Hubbard

Poor   **Good**

Excellent

NON-STARCHY VEGETABLES
(high water-content foods)

Asparagus	Eggplant	Radishes*
Beet Greens	Endive	Scallions*
Broccoli	Escarole	Spinach
Brussles Sprouts	Garlic	Sprouts
Cabbage	Green Beans	Squash
Celery	Kale	Sweet Pepper
Chard	Kohlrabi	Swiss Chard
Chicory	Leeks*	Tomatoes
Collards	Lettuce	Turnips
Cucumber	Onions*	Watercress
Dandelion	Parsley	Zucchini

Excellent   **Excellent**

Good   **Good**

MILDLY-STARCHY VEGETABLES

Artichokes	Carrots	Corn
Beets	Cauliflower	Peas

Known irritants should be eaten sparingly or not at all

ACID FRUIT

Blackberry	Plum (Sour)
Grapefruit	Pomegranete
Lemon/Lime	Raspberry
Orange	Sour Apple
Pineapple	Strawberry

SUB-ACID FRUIT

Apple	Mango
Apricot	Papaya
Blueberry	Peach
Cherry	Pear
Kiwi	Plum (sweet)

SWEET FRUIT

Banana	Grapes
Dates	Papaya
Currents	Persimmon
Figs	Prunes
Fruit, Dried	Raisins

MELON

Cantaloupe	Papaya
Casaba	Persian
Crenshaw	Musk
Honeydew	Watermeon

- Only eat fruit alone as a fruit meal
- Food should not be eaten between meals while other food is digesting in the stomach

- Do not est sweet fruits and acid fruits together
- Melons are best eaten alone but can be mixed with Acid and sub-acid fruits

Washing

Statistics show that anywhere from 9 to 48 million people get sick from dirty food every year.[61] We can easily defend against these illnesses by washing our produce before eating. Even a 20 second water rinse will get rid of some of the bacteria that may be accompanying your food. Leafy greens carry the most toxin agents, so be mindful to wash them thoroughly.

2 Recipes for Homemade Food Washes:[62]

1. 1 Tablespoon lemon juice
   2 Tablespoons distilled white vinegar
   1 cup cold tap water in a spray bottle
   Spray on food and then be sure to rinse off afterwards.

2. 1 cup distilled white vinegar 3 cups water
   Mix the water and vinegar together in a bowl. Allow your greens to soak in the bowl for about 2 minutes, then rinse them well.

This #2 wash, which researchers from the magazine *Cook's Illustrated* found killed 98 percent of bacteria on food. It is good for leafy greens because greens are more likely than other forms of produce to be contaminated with E. coli bacteria, according to the CDC. If you want even more of the germ-killing boost, add a tablespoon or two of salt. A study in the *Journal of Food Protection* found that vinegar's ability to kill E. coli bacteria was "significantly enhanced" when salt was added to the mix.

Sprouting[63]

Nuts, seeds, grains and legumes are high in vitamins and minerals; and they are at their most beneficial when sprouted. Basically, the nutrition

---

61 http://healthyeating.sfgate.com/clean-fruits-vegetables-vinegar-8777.html http://www.rodalenews.com/veggie-wash

62 Excerpt taken directly from: http://www.rodalenews.com/veggie-wash http://www.trueactivist.com/6-food-combining-rules-for-optimal-digestion/ http://mostlyraw.eu/2011/07/12/introduction-to-food-combining/

63 For products and information visit: http://sproutpeople.org/seeds/

in these foods is inactive until they start to germinate. This means they need to be soaked in order to derive their maximum benefit. Once they are germinated we are eating more than just a seed, we are eating a tiny plant, which is loaded with all the good stuff.

Seeds, legumes and grains contain phytic acid and enzyme inhibitors, which render them inactive, blocking much of their nutritional value. When we soak and sprout them these inhibitors are broken down making the calcium, magnesium, iron, copper, zinc and other vitamins and minerals accessible to humans. Without sprouting they are very hard to digest and can cause bloating and gas.

Once active they become powerhouses for nutrition. Vitamin A, B, C, D, E, K, Amino acids, and trace elements to name a few become active and readily available. Some research suggests that the bioavailability of protein can increase 35%.[64]

Alternatives

Below are alternative food suggestions for some regularly consumed foods. They are delicious and provide more nutritional value for your body. Try them and see how they make you feel.

1. A tasty and nutritious substitute for dairy milk is almond, hemp or coconut milk.
2. Try nutritional yeast on pasta or for making a pesto instead of cheese.
3. Nuts and seeds are better snacks than crackers or chips. I like the GoRaw and Living Intentions companies because they sprout and season their nuts.
4. Apple cider vinegar is an alkalizing alternative to balsamic vinegar.
5. Coconut water, kombucha, herbal teas, or green tea in place of soda or coffee.
6. Try sorbet instead of ice cream. Coconut ice cream is delicious.
7. Use honey or raw agave in place of sugar. In smoothies, dates, raisins and goji berries can all be used as sweetening agents.

64   http://www.thenourishinggourmet.com/2009/01/why-sprout.html

Soaking and Sprouting Times

Nut / Seed	Dry Amount	Soak Time	Sprout Time	Sprout Length	Yield
Alfalfa Seed	3 Tbsp	12 Hours	3-5 Days	1-2 Inches	4 Cups
Almonds	3 Cups	8-12 Hours	1-3 Days	1/8 Inch	4 Cups
Amaranth	1 Cup	3-5 Hours	2-3 Days	1/4 Inch	3 Cups
Barley - Hulless	1 Cup	6 Hours	12-24 Hours	1/4 Inch	2 Cups
Broccoli Seed	2 Tbsp	8 Hours	3-4 Days	1-2 Inches	2 Cups
Buckwheat - Hulled	1 Cup	6 Hours	1-2 Days	1/8-1/2 Inch	2 Cups
Cabbage Seed	1 Tbsp	4-6 Hours	4-5 Days	1-2 Inches	1 1/2 Cups
Cashews	3 Cups	2-3 Hours			4 Cups
Clover	3 Tbsp	5 Hours	4-6 Days	1-2 Inches	4 Cups
Fenugreek	4 Tbsp	6 Hours	2-5 Days	1-2 Inches	3 Cups
Flax Seeds	1 Cup	6 Hours			2 Cups
Chick Peas	1 Cup	12-48 Hours	2-4 Days	1/2-1 Inch	4 Cups
Kale Seed	4 Tbsp	4-6 Hours	4-6 Days	3/4-1 Inch	3-4 Cups
Lentil	3/4 Cup	8 Hours	2-3 Days	1/2-1 Inch	4 Cups
Millet	1 Cup	5 Hours	12 Hours	1/16 Inch	3 Cups
Mung Beans	1/3 Cup	8 Hours	4-5 Days	1/4-3 Inches	4 Cups
Mustard Seed	3 Tbsp	5 Hours	3-5 Days	1/2-1 1/2 Inches	3 Cups
Oats, Hulled	1 Cup	8 Hours	1-2 Days	1/8 Inch	1 Cup
Onion Seed	1 Tbsp	4-6 Hours	4-5 Days	1-2 Inches	1 1/2-2 Cups
Pea	1 Cup	8 Hours	2-3 Days	1/2-1 Inch	3 Cups
Pinto Bean	1 Cup	12 Hours	3-4 Days	1/2-1 Inch	3-4 Cups
Pumpkin	1 Cup	6 Hours	1-2 Days	1/8 Inch	2 Cups
Quinoa	1 Cup	3-4 Hours	2-3 Days	1/2 Inch	3 Cups
Radish	3 Tbsp	6 Hours	3-5 Days	3/4-2 Inches	4 Cups
Rye	1 Cup	6-8 Hours	2-3 Days	1/2-3/4 Inch	3 Cups
Sesame Seed - Hulled	1 Cup	8 Hours			1 1/2 Cups
Sesame Seed - Unhulled	1 Cup	4-6 Hours	1-2 Days	1/8 Inch	1 Cup
Spelt	1 Cup	6 Hours	1-2 Days	1/4 Inch	3 Cups
Sunflower - Hulled	1 Cup	6-8 Hours	1 Day	1/4-1/2 Inch	2 Cups
Teff	1 Cup	3-4 Hours	1-2 Days	1/8 Inch	3 Cups
Walnuts	3 Cups	4 Hours			4 Cups
Wheat	1 Cup	8-10 Hours	2-3 Days	1/4-3/4 Inch	3 Cups
Wild Rice	1 Cup	12 Hours	2-3 Days	Rice Splits	3 Cups

8. Bragg's Liquid Aminos is a delicious and healthy substitute for soy sauce.

9. Use Celtic or Himalayan sea salt in place of table salt.

10. Nut "cheeses" are healthy and tasty alternatives to dairy cheese. Check www.dr-cow.com.

11. For bread, make sure to buy sprouted grains. I like the Ezekiel Company for this very reason.

12. Try hummus, salsa and guacamole in place of creamy, cheesy and oily dips.

13. There are many white flour pasta alternatives on the market now like spirulina, quinoa, black bean and rice pastas as well as kelp noodles.

In a Sprouted Nut Shell
Nut Shell 1 — Julian's Ultra-Brief Summary

Noted below are some simple and general guidelines for maximizing your health potential:

1. Drink lots of water.

2. Eat fresh, local, seasonal, colorful, organic food. Lots of dark leafy greens. You can find these products at the farmers market or on the periphery of the supermarket.

3. Reduce or eliminate caffeine and sodas.

4. Limit sugar and eliminate artificial sweeteners.

5. Eat superfoods.

6. Avoid pesticides.

7. Eat quality animal protein.

8. Sprout nuts and seeds.

9. Use small plates when dishing out your food to reduce over-consumption. Eat slowly, preferably with others and without background distractions like the television.

10. Cook your own food.

11. The book, *Hungry for Health*, by Susan Silberstein, Ph.D. outlines 4 principles for eating healthy: 1) Eat Primitive; 2) Eat Colorful; 3) Eat Alkaline; 4) Eat Organic.

12. Michael Pollan's guidelines from *In Defense of Food*: 1) Eat Food; 2) Mostly Plants; 3) Not too Much.

Nut Shell 2 — Suggestions from the Sonne's Company for General Health Enhancement

Victor Earl Irons is the founder of the Sonne's Organic Food, Inc., a legendary nutritionist and health freedom fighter. At age 40 he was diagnosed with severe ankylosing spondylitis, an arthritic condition that causes the formation of calcium deposits along the spine. Many doctors told him there was no cure. In 14 months, by using natural methods and no drugs, he defied all odds and cured himself. He went on to lecture across the country and develop natural vitamins that have been helping people for over 60 years. He founded the National Health Federation, which helped to push bills through Congress that allowed for natural vitamins not to be banned by the FDA. The Sonne's mission statement is:

Our mission is to educate the consumer on matters of nutrition and health, empowering you and your families with the knowledge to make the right decisions about the foods you eat and the consequences they have.[65]

Below is a list of recommendations for healthy eating and lifestyle that come directly from Sonne's:

Dos

1. Eat a raw vegetable salad daily — eat it before starting the main course.
2. Eat two or more pieces of **fresh fruit daily**.
3. Eat **fruits** only for dessert, preferable raw.
4. Use **concentrated proteins** only once daily — less concentrated proteins anytime.

---

65   For more information check out: http://sonnes.com

5. **Cook** beef on the rare side, eggs soft, and vegetables as raw as possible.
6. **Drink** water heavily between meals - but not for two hours after or half-hour before.
7. **Melons** are best eaten between meals.
8. Eat a large helping of cooked **leafy vegetable** daily - for laxative purposes.
9. "**Eat nothing unless it will spoil** or **rot** but eat it before it does." — Dr. McCollum
10. **Exercise** — even well balanced blood is ineffective unless aerated (oxygenated) so walk, walk, walk!
11. Condition the mind with **positive thinking**.

Don'ts

1. **Don't** drink **milk** and eat **meat** at the same meal. Although milk is a Protein, it requires a different digestive medium than concentrated proteins like meat, fish and poultry. The old Mosaic Law made it a sin to drink milk with meat. Avoid building toxic **poisons** of **undigested proteins** when meat and milk are used at the same meal since neither may properly digest. **Use milk as the only protein of the meal, and not as a beverage** with meat.
2. Eliminate from the diet all products made of refined, white or whole wheat bleached and chemically treated flours synthetically fortified. These "empty calorie" products merely take the place of truly nutritious foods. Use products made from unbleached flour, which still contains its nutritional value. If your intestinal tract can take it use whole grain flours.
3. **Eliminate all refined sugars** and all products presweetened when purchased. They are usually sweetened with white sugar and/or synthetic glucose, which again merely supply "empty calories." Use only honey, maple syrup, raw or dark brown sugar and unsulphured molasses.

4. **Never cook anything** you can possibly eat **raw**.

5. Never eat **desserts** — except **fruits**.

6. **Avoid** all **meats** treated with **synthetic hormones** or **chemicals**.

7. **Avoid** all **fats** that have been "hydrogenated."

Chapter 5

Purification Practices (Cleanses)

If the doors of perception were cleansed everything
would appear to man as it is, infinite.
—William Blake

What is a cleanse?

A cleanse is a generic term for anything you do to limit toxic intake and assist your body in ridding itself of stored toxicity. Some people simply eliminate one thing from their diet such as sugar. Others use herbs, colon hydrotherapy or go to a detoxification center or retreat to have a deeper experience. This section will focus specifically on the body. Cleanses can include, but are not limited to, our mind and emotions, our physical space and lifestyle choices or relationships.

Cleansing is all the craze nowadays. It is more common now than ever to hear that someone is cleansing. So what is it that everyone is doing? How are they doing it? What are the steps to successfully completing a cleanse? Why cleanse?

The history behind cleansing is quite long. Since the beginning of recorded history people across the world have been using a plethora of techniques for body purification. Panchakarma is a traditional form of Indian cleansing, which consists of massage, herbal compounds, colon cleansing, specified diets and mental exercises. It can last anywhere from 1 week to months, most are a minimum of 3 weeks. The Chinese have the first written herbal prescriptions dating back to 2700 BCE. Colon hydrotherapy, also known as colonics, was first recorded in 1500 BCE, and sauna has been used since the year 1112 as a form of cleansing.[1]

The philosophies behind cleansing are as vast and varied as its history. Cleansing is an experiment to see what works and what does not. Not all cleanses are for all people. The suggestions listed here are cleansing practices that can be built into your everyday lifestyles. They are aimed at maximizing the body's own detoxification capacity and assist in the correction of toxin related ailments.

Even though the focus of this section is on the body, the purification process can reveal more than just physical toxicity. Unhealthy emotional, mental and spiritual patterning can surface. These awarenesses are just as important as the physical process. Be mindful and pay close attention to what you feel and think as your body is cleansed.

The Basics
Organs of Elimination and Detoxification

Though every cell of the body plays an important role in detoxification, there are organs that specialize in "waste management."[2] A brief discussion about the key organs of detoxification will give us a base understanding of how our incredible human machine works. These major organs and ways to assist them during the initial detoxification are as follows:

---

1 http://www.aviva.ca/article.asp?articleid=102#ixzz2wA7Ytq3e

2 The organ metaphors, represented in "", throughout this section come from: *The Golden Bridge Yogi's Cleanse Manual for Transformation and Rejuvenation*. Grace and gratitude to the author of this work.

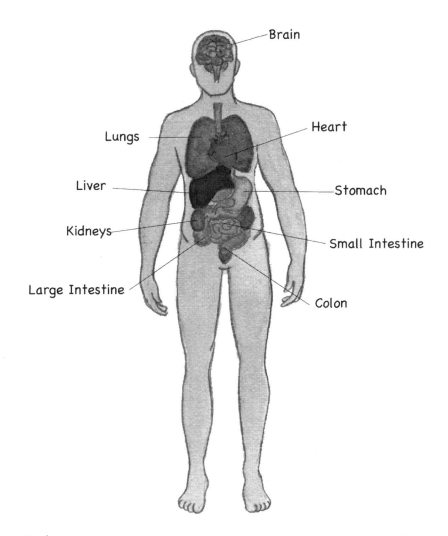

Colon The colon is our "solid waste management" organ in the body. It plays an essential role in the final stages of digestion and elimination. Many people have thick mucous linings, rubber-like waste and putrefied matter stuck in the walls of the colon (and intestines). Most weight is lost through the colon.

Colon hydrotherapy, enemas and implants are highly effective practices for cleaning the colon of stuck matter.

Gut Microbiome Our gut microbiome or microbiota refers to the communities of bacteria that live in our bodies. In some Eastern wisdom traditions, they believed that millions of deities live in our bellies — perhaps they clued into the gut bacteria. In fact, there are trillions of bacteria. They play a vital role in our mental, emotional and physical health. Everything from our brain to our immune system is impacted by the health of our *gut bugs*.[3] Scientists and researchers are now studying the importance of gut health.[4]

Kidneys The "water management" organs. The kidneys are responsible for keeping the chemistry of the blood alkaline by filtering out the dissolved acid wastes. In Traditional Chinese Medicine (TCM), the kidneys are your battery pack, representing willpower and energy levels. TCM also suggests that the kidneys are linked to fear emotion.

Fresh water and juices help power the kidneys during cleanses.

Liver The "recycling center." This organ has over 200 functions in the body. It is the main player in detoxification by sorting out the toxins, breaking them down and expelling them from the body. In TCM, the liver correlates with the anger emotion and can be regulated with self-acceptance.

A balanced acid/alkaline diet, exercise, and proper hydration help assist the liver during detoxification.

Lungs The blood's "air purifiers." The lungs are the main organ in your respiratory system. They bring fresh oxygen into the bloodstream, while filtering out toxins from the air, they also remove waste gases that are produced by the body's cells. In TCM, the lungs represent the grief and integrity/dignity emotions.

Deep breathing helps keep the blood alkaline which is most important for maintaining and health organism. See the breathing section for helpful exercises. In short, breathe deeply to activate movement of the diaphragm.

Lymph The major "cleansing channels" in the body. They are an intricate network of tubing that carries the bulk of waste and toxicity from the cells to the final elimination organs. Major lymphatic glands (holding tanks) are the appendix, spleen, thymus and tonsils. These glands may tend to swell during detoxification. In TCM, the lymph system is governed by the spleen and correlates with the worry and trust emotions.

3 A term often used by Dr. Perlmutter in *Brain Maker*

4 For more information check out The National Institutes of Health — Human Microbiome Project: Bhttps://commonfund.nih.gov/hmp/

The lymphatic system does not move on its own and therefore requires help from exercise, massage and proper hydration. Laughter also helps move the lymphatic system, so throw on your favorite comedy and laugh your way to health.

Skin The "temperature/humidity controller." The skin is the body's largest organ and plays a key role in the elimination of toxic agents. In addition to regulating temperature and body moisture content, the skin often functions as a backup for the other elimination organs. In TCM, the skin is linked to the functioning of the lungs.

Exercise, sweating, skin brushing, massage, and hydration all encourage healthy skin and the elimination of toxicity.

Key Concepts for Optimal Detoxification

1. **Investigate** Identify and get rid of toxins. We live in a modern world that has tremendous amounts of toxicity. After the industrial revolution and with the continued use of chemicals to treat our land and food, we now have higher rates of disease causing agents than ever before. By minimizing our contact with these agents, we can live a healthier life. This means that we must investigate our body, as it as, and make better choices for what we put into it.

2. **Purify** Purify your body. The source of toxic load for many is in the gut. This is not the only place where toxins live, but where much of it is processed. By making simple adjustments to our diet we can begin to purify naturally. Creating a balanced acid/alkaline environment for our body is one of the best ways to combat any current or potential disease.

3. **Movement** A simple truth about human existence is that movement is nonnegotiable. By exercising, we encourage the oxygenation of our cells, the delivery of nutrients and expulsion of toxicity. Many of the toxins in our body are stored in our fat cells, so by exercising, we can purge these unfriendlies. Unlike our breath, our lymphatic system does not move automatically. By moving

our body, we activate our lymphatic system and increase overall circulation.

4. **Support** Support the body and mind their natural detoxification process. With proper guidance we can build the necessary environment for maximum detoxification. Organic foods and superfoods, vitamin and herbal supplementation, exercise, body-work and group support are all components of supporting the body and mind.

5. **The Nonphysical** Detoxify mind, heart and spirit. We are multi-dimensional beings and must work on cleansing other parts of our self as well. By investigating our mental, emotional and spiritual parts, we can uncover many other areas that will aid and facilitate this process. This is one of the most important parts of the process because mental/emotional stress is the leading cause of disease in our lives.[5]

Tips For Optimal Physical Detoxifications

1. **Set Intentions** Consider these questions: 1) Why am I cleansing? 2) What do I want to gain from this experience? 3) What are some of my fears? Consider, contemplate and write what comes to mind.

2. **Seek Guidance** Consult your physician or experienced cleanse leader before taking on any cleanse to see if it is right for you. Depending on your symptoms, genetic predispositions and environmental exposures, you may need different levels of nutrients and types of treatment. With support you can go much deeper.

3. **Drink Water** 3-4 liters of water, depending on your weight and how much you exercise (refer to p. 62-64).

4. **Poop** The colon is a major component to the detoxification (and weight loss) process. Enemas, colon hydrotherapy, and herbs can

---

5   CDC suggests that 80% of all dollars spent on illness in America are stress related. Bruce Lipton suggests that 95% of illness is due to stress.

help aid in healthy movements. If you are a bit "stuck," drink more water and fresh juice and/or eat more fibrous fruits and vegetables. Regular exercise also helps your bowels.

5. **E.A.T.** (refer to p. 61-88) Eat as much local, organic and seasonal produce as possible — eight to ten servings of colorful fruits and vegetables daily. Eliminate all animal products, processed food, soda, alcohol, tobacco, stimulants, sedatives, drugs, caffeine, white flour and refined sugars.

6. **Exercise** By conditioning your cardiovascular system with strengthening and stretching exercises, the body can detoxify more efficiently and rejuvenate faster. Start by adding 10-15 minutes of walk to your daily regiment. Incorporate stretching as much as possible – perhaps in front of the television. If you are motivated, hire a personal trainer, join and gym or find a sports league near you. Do something you enjoy doing, but move your body everyday.

7. **Sweat** Use a sauna, steam or a detoxification bath in order to clean and open the pores of the skin. In Europe, saunas are commonplace. It is a practice that has been happening for thousands of years. Saunas can help with fatigue, mild depression, arthritis, muscular pain, skin conditions and promote cardiovascular flow.[6]

8. **Relax** Cleansing can induce bodily changes in which rest and relaxation are tremendously beneficial. Try mediating, deep breathing, or your favorite relaxation technique.

9. **Educate** Read something on health and nutrition to educate yourself on your mind, body and/or spirit. The "Recommended Reading" section offers a list of books and media for your enjoyment.

10. **Bodywork** This is the time to indulge in massage, acupuncture, chiropractic or energy work. Find a practitioner near you and spoil yourself.

---

6 http://www.drwhitaker.com/health-benefits-of-a-sauna

Healing Crisis

During the detoxification process, many people experience what is called a "healing crisis." Healing crises can manifest in many different ways: nausea, dizziness, tiredness, achiness, headaches, restlessness and emotional outbursts. This is an indicator that the process is working (if you do not experience a healing crisis, it is ok, the process is still working). If and when this happens, remember to take it easy — rest, relax and take it slow.

When we allow our body to detoxify much of what is stored gets released — enjoy the physical restructuring. We must allow our organs to do their jobs, even if that means not feeling good for a few days. Afterwards, it is normal to experience a surge of energy, increased clarity, sustained stamina and improved sensitivity to foods.

Purify

Below are a few techniques for purification that are inexpensive, effective and easy. Try them and notice what happens.

The Mouth and Tongue

The mouth is home to millions of bacteria, including streptococcus mutans, which can cause cavities, gingivitis, plaque, tooth decay, bad breath and other more menacing illnesses. Cleaning the mouth is one of the most basic and easiest forms of purification. In the US, we take great care of our teeth by brushing, flossing, and using mouthwash. It is so mainstream that we do not even consider it a cleanse, but it is! In Thailand, it is a cultural tradition to routinely wash hands, feet and mouth. In India, oil pulling (see below) is another standard daily practice that helps to promote a healthy mouth.

In Chinese medicine, the tongue is used as an indicator for overall health in the body. A brief examination by a doctor can inform them on what might be happening deeper inside. In the Basilica of St. Anthony in Padua, Italy they have preserved St. Anthony's tongue. He was known

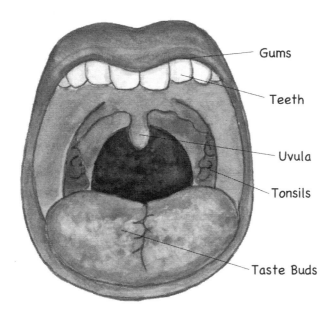

Gums

Teeth

Uvula

Tonsils

Taste Buds

for his powerful preaching and is often prayed to for finding lost things or people. In the tradition of Ayurveda, people massage or scrape their tongues with the belief that they will become better public speakers, be more mindful with their words and can express themselves by sincerely speaking from the heart.

According to Kundalini Yoga teacher and prenatal expert, Gurmukh, the tongue is the second muscle to begin to form during the development of a baby in utero (the first being the heart). Have you ever heard the expression, "speak from the heart?" This could be the origin of such statements. Gurmukh, while studying with yogis in India, learned the practice of tongue massaging. This practice can trigger thousands of physical, mental and spiritual functions. It is a good way to practice the notion of speaking compassionately from the heart.

To speak from the heart with pearly white teeth and fresh breath (or if you just want a clean mouth), try oil pulling and tongue scraping.

Two techniques for cleaning the mouth and tongue:

Oil pulling

Oil pulling is simple and suggested to be done daily. Bacteria is fat-soluble so by introducing fatty oils, the bacteria gets pulled from the body and consumed by the oil. This removal helps our body with its natural functions of cleaning the mouth first. This practice has been shown to help with cavities, gingivitis and tooth decay. In 2008, a study[7] showed that significant lowering of bacteria in the mouth with the use of coconut oil. In another study, at the Athlone Institute of Technology's Bioscience Research Institute in Ireland, Dr. Damien Brady said:

> Incorporating enzyme-modified coconut oil into dental hygiene products would be an attractive alternative to chemical additives, particularly as it works at relatively low concentrations. Also, with increasing antibiotic resistance, it is important that we turn our attention to new ways to combat microbial infection.[8]

Try this practice and notice the benefits. It is also an easy way to enjoy in Noble Silence (by not having to speak with anyone — great for the morning).

DIRECTIONS:

1. Take a heaping teaspoon of coconut oil or sesame seed oil, put it in your mouth and slosh it around for about 20 minutes without swallowing.
2. After 20 minutes, spit out the oil. Be mindful to spit the oil outside or in a receptacle designated for oil. This can clog drains, corrode pipes and be detrimental to the public water systems.

Tongue Cleaning/Scraping

The power of the tongue is recognized in many traditions; so that maintaining its health is critical for *robust vitality*.

A tongue cleaner or tongue scraper is another inexpensive yet transformative tool that is highly recommended for body purification. A typical tongue scraper is a thin, u-shaped piece of stainless steel (a spoon will work as well) removes plaque, bacteria and leftover food particles

---

7 http://www.ncbi.nlm.nih.gov/pubmed/18408265

8 http://articles.mercola.com/sites/articles/archive/2012/12/08/coconut-oil-combats-tooth-decay.aspx

from the surface of the tongue. Use a tongue cleaner to fight cavities, gingivitis and tooth decay.

Another added benefit of tongue scraping is the reduction of cravings. By cleaning away any leftover food the body is less apt to crave the foods previously eaten. A tongue scraper can actually make your tongue more alive by stimulating its taste buds. When old residue, bacteria and food particles are removed from the tongue, our quality of taste enhances making all food more pleasurable to consume.

Note: Using a toothbrush for this technique helps, but is not as useful as a tongue scraper. Brushing the tongue with a toothbrush does move things around but does not get the deep clean that a tongue scraper does.

DIRECTIONS:

1. Use the rounded cleaning edge to scrape gently down the tongue several times, while applying slight pressure. The pressure applied to the tongue is firm, but not hard - this process should not induce pain. Do two to three times per day, in the shower, after brushing your teeth, or in between meals. Rinse and repeat until there is no white residue left on the tongue.

Neti Pot
– written by Katy Cox

The Neti pot has been used since ancient times as an effective aid keep nasal and sinus passages clear of excess mucus and calm inflammation caused by allergies and infections. These little pots can be made from Plastic, terracotta or metal and are commonly used by yogis to clear the nasal passages before they yoga asana and pranayama. Ear, nose, and throat surgeons recommend nasal irrigation with a Neti pot, or other irrigation method, for their patients who've undergone sinus surgery, to clear away crusting in the nasal passages. Many people with sinus symptoms from allergies and environmental irritants also have begun to regularly use the Neti pot or other nasal irrigation devices, claiming that these devices alleviate congestion, and facial pain and pressure. Research backs up these claims, finding that nasal irrigation can be an effective way to relieve sinus symptoms. For some people, nasal irrigation may bring relief of sinus symptoms without the use of medications.

Typically the neti pot is filled with 16Oz of warm **filtered water** (not tap water), to which 1tsp of **Sea salt** is added. The nozzle of the neti is then placed gently inside the nostril to seal it and the head tipped to 45 degree angle. The fluid flows through the nasal cavity and out the other side. It may also run into the throat from where it should be spat out. Getting the correct tilt of the head takes a little practice but soon becomes easy and, some find, pleasurable to perform. Use a full neti for each nostril, taking time to stop and clear each nostril thoroughly by blowing gently until any mucus is expelled. Please ask if you would like a demonstration or to try the neti for yourself.

Gentle Internal Cleanse With Apple Cider Vinegar
– written by Katy Cox

Organic Apple Cider Vinegar is a detoxifying antioxidant that breaks up blockages in the body and has been shown to lower blood sugar level and cholesterol. It is full of antibiotic properties that can rebalance the acid content in your stomach, preventing heartburn and acid reflex. Drinking just a cap full in the morning helps to cleanse the colon (helping that to clear that indigestion that might have cause the residue on your tongue from our above practice). Just be sure that you buy the organic unfiltered version.

The vinegar also stimulates your metabolism and digestion for the day, preparing your body for balanced energy use and even weight loss. I recommend adding the capful in a big glass of water and drinking the whole thing down first thing in the morning. If the taste is too much for you, you can even heat the water a little and mix in a teaspoon of honey. Just a spoonful helps the medicine go down!

Besides taking Apple Cider Vinegar internally, it has a myriad of topical uses. If you have problems with a rash, acne, bug bites or poison ivy, just put some Apple Cider Vinegar on it. Using ACV as a final rinse for the hair leaves it soft and shiny and can help control dandruff and excess oil production. The vinegar is also effective in cleaning, from counters to sterilizing, this is your chemical-free go to!

Colon Cleanse

Cleaning the colon is very important for the process of detoxification. As mentioned above, the colon is our waste management system. It is also the last phase of digestion assimilating any unprocessed nutrients into the body. It is important that we keep this area of our body clean and functioning at its highest capability. In some Eastern cultures, the health of their elderly is measured by the strength and efficiency of the colon. Outside of colon hydrotherapy and enemas (which I highly recommend), the saltwater flush is a useful technique for clearing any blockages.

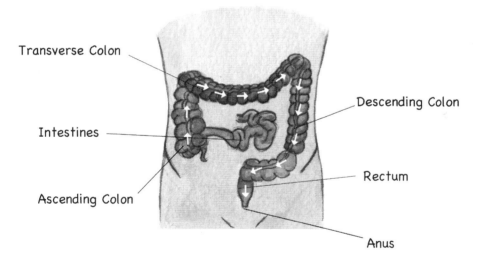

Salt Water Flush The salt-water flush is used to stimulate bowel movements and eliminate waste from the colon. The salt in the water simulates the same gravity as human blood and therefore passes through the kidneys and processes its way out internally cleansing the entire way. Do this practice in the morning on an empty stomach. It is simple, effective, relatively painless and acts very quickly. It can be just as effective as a colonic and is an important addition to any juice or water fast.

DIRECTIONS:

1. Take 1 tablespoon of sea salt and add it to 1 quart of warm (preferably) water. Drink this solution in 30 minutes or less. Sea salt is highly recommended for this process because it carries more minerals than regular iodized table Salt. Do not use Epsom salt it can be too corrosive.

2. Try not to eat for approximately 2 hours and be near a bathroom.

3. If it does not work, adjust the amount of salt that you put in the water.

Diatomaceous Earth
– written by Katy Cox

Diatomaceous earth is a white organic powder, which technically comes from the cell walls of fossilized single-cell diatoms — essentially, it's a fossil, ground into a very fine powder. There are two general types of diatomaceous earth: food grade and industrial grade. While industrial grade is toxic to humans and pets, food grade diatomaceous earth is non-toxic and very beneficial on multiple levels

When viewed through a microscope, it looks like a hollow cylinder, with holes throughout the side. It carries a strong negative charge. If you'll recall your science lessons, you'll remember that negatively charged ions are attracted to positively charged ions. Therefore, when taken internally, the diatomaceous earth attracts and absorbs positively-charged pathogens into its cylinder — it absorbs the things we want to stay away from, like viruses, pathogenic fungi and bacteria, heavy metals, prescription drug residues, pesticides, parasites, radiation, and the like — and sweeps them out of our bodies. As this powder makes its way through our digestive tract, it gently "scrubs" the packed-on residue we have there and sweeps it out of our bodies. Nice, diatoms!

Also, because of this quality, it is very sharp. Organisms such as parasites, lurking in our intestines, are sliced up and killed, and swept away when we empty our bowels, and we are left unharmed.

The last quality I'll mention is also powerful: food grade diatomaceous earth is 84% silica, and contains some 20 trace minerals. Did you know life can't exist without silica? It is essential for the building of healthy bones and teeth, skin, hair, and nails. As our mineral resources are getting depleted, our food is containing less and less silica. Do yourself a favor and add this divine diatom to your diet.

To take diatomaceous earth, all you have to do is mix a spoonful into some water or other liquid, and drink. Follow with another cup of water. (Diatomaceous earth can make you thirsty — make sure and drink plenty of water while using this supplement.) It's that easy! You can also add it to smoothies — it's totally undetected that way.

Dosage: If you are just beginning your diatomaceous earth journey, start with a teaspoon mixed in liquid, as I've detailed above, once a day, Before bed being an optimal time. Slowly increase the amount taken, up to a heaping tablespoon, and up to three times a day.

Diatomaceous earth is a way to detox your body, and if you start with too much, your body will get rid of toxins too quickly and leave you feeling under the weather. Yes, it really does work that well! If you start experiencing slight headaches, you'll know you took it a little fast. But don't stop altogether, just do yourself a favor and **take it slowly** — no need to rush.

Body Scrubbing

Body scrubbing is an ancient holistic practice that many cultures have used to help purify their skin and entire body. In ancient Rome, bones were used to scrub the skin at bathhouses. In present day Morocco, they enjoy what's called *hammam*, which includes bathing and body scrubbing. Some traditions use honey or different essential oils to help exfoliate the skin. Cleansing the skin and clearing the pores is nothing new, so why is it so important?

The skin is the largest organ in the body and is an important organ for detoxification because it breathes — in traditional Chinese medicine it is related to the lungs (and large intestines). Its pores help expel toxins and assimilate nutrients from the exterior. By body scrubbing we stimulate the pores, improve circulation, encourage the lymphatic system, and induce a general feeling of goodness.

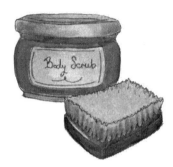

Body scrubbing can be done before or after your bathing or anytime during the day. There are several different techniques that can be applied. A hot towel, scrub brush, or even using your nails are all effective means of scrubbing. For the maximum effect, scrub your body twice a day: once in the morning and once in the evening outside of the shower. Enjoy scrubbing for (at least) 2 to 20 minutes.

BENEFITS:
1. Reduces muscle tension.
2. Opens the pores to release stored toxins.
3. Encourages excess fat, mucus, and toxins to discharge rather than to accumulate around deeper vital organs.
4. Relieves stress.
5. Calms the mind.
6. Promotes circulation.
7. Activates the lymphatic system, especially when scrubbing under-arms and groin.
8. It is an easy way to self-care.

This can be a sacred moment in your day if done with loving affection and proper intention, especially by showing love and affection for body parts that are usually neglected.

Hot Towel Scrub

DIRECTIONS:

1. Fill the sink with hot water.
2. Soak towel/washcloth in the hot water and ring it out.
3. While the towel is hot scrub the skin gently.
4. Do one section of the body at a time, rinsing the towel/washcloth as often as you like keeping it warm and fresh. Scrub the entire body from head to toe and everywhere in between.
5. Scrub until the skin becomes slightly pink or until each part becomes warm.

Scrub Brush/Glove

DIRECTIONS:

1. Take brush/glove and gently scrub the entire body.
2. Use circular motions.
3. Take care to scrub in between your legs and under your armpits.

Homemade Body Scrub[9]

INGREDIENTS:

1/2 cup + 2 tablespoons Epsom salt or coarse salt crystals.

2 tablespoons of olive oil.

Juice of one lemon or lime .

Herb of choice (optional).

Combine all the ingredients, adding the lemon last and put them in a sealed container. Scrub 2 times per week. You can do this before, during or after a shower. If after, make sure to rinse off.

Heavy Metal Removal

Removing heavy metals is key for optimal health. Heavy metal toxicity can cause many illnesses from cancer to fatigue, sinus problems

---

9 http://everydayroots.com/homemade-body-scrub-recipe Consult these websites for more body scrub ideas: http://www.treehugger.com/organic-beauty/8-homemade-salt-and-sugar-body-scrubs.html http://mashable.com/2014/07/20/homemade-body-scrubs/

to allergies, headaches to a wide array of digestion issues. Common culprits are the metal amalgam fillings[10] in your teeth. From my personal experience and observing others that have had their fillings removed the results are tremendous. Less sickness, more energy, and greater mental clarity are but a few of the benefits. If you do have metal amalgam fillings, I strongly sug- gest you get them removed and replaced immediately.

Note: Find a dentist that has experience in this practice because the process is very particular. Check http://www.nihadc.com to find someone near you.

In the mean time, there are certain foods and herbs that can help to slowly encapsulate and move the metals out. Chlorella, a single-celled, freshwater algae, is known to bind to heavy metals, particularly mercury, and can help usher them out of the body. Cilantro is also a useful herb to help with this process as well. In combination with chlorella, the cilantro is best taken about 45 minutes after the chlorella and in warm water.

Bentonite clay is another nature aid for the elimination of heavy metals. It is an aged volcanic ash that bonds to heavy metals, then releases its minerals (high in silica, magnesium, sodium, iron, potassium). It helps to oxygenate and alkalize the body.[11]

Lastly, heavy metal chelation therapy is a highly effective practice that I have embraced over the past several years. It requires intravenous injections of particular agents that are excellent at removing metals from your body. You will be monitored by doctors and can see your progress with frequent testing. I have seen tremendous benefits, such as allergy elimination, more energy, better sleep patterns and increased cognitive function.

---

10 The National Integrated Health Associates, NIHA is Washington, D.C. is a tremendous resource for finding qualified practitioners for metal amalgam removal and chelation therapy. http://www.nihadc.com

11 Arizona State did a study that found bentonite clay effective in killing salmonella, e.coli. (http://wellnessmama.com/5915/the-benefits-of- healing-clays/)

Tips for Reducing Your
Intake of Heavy Metals[12]

1. Avoid consuming deep-sea fish like tuna, mackerel and swordfish. Shellfish like oysters, clams and lobster also carry high levels of heavy metals.
2. Drink purified water because much of our public water supply has been contaminated.
3. Use stainless steel or glass instead of aluminum pots and pans.
4. Avoid using aluminum foil or drinking out of aluminum cans.
5. Get your fillings removed.
6. E.A.T. organic whole foods.

Bath, Body and Skincare Products

What we put on our body is just as important as what goes in (and what is eliminated). Many of the body and beauty care products that are on the market today could actually be making us sick. Our skin is porous and therefore absorbs a lot of what we put on it. Taking the proper care to avoid certain ingredients is a valuable asset in our overall health. Sunscreens, soap, shampoo, and body lotions are all worthy of further investigation.

Things to Avoid[13]

1. **Parabens:** Found in makeup, bodywash, deodorants, and shampoos. Suspected endocrine disruptor, associated with increased risk of breast cancer and may interfere with male reproductive system.

12 For more information on Heavy Metal precautions check out: http://naturopathconnect.com/articles/heavy-metal-toxicity-dietary/ and http://www.hugginsappliedhealing.com

13 useful links: http://www.mindbodygreen.com/0-5971/12-Toxic-Ingredients-to-AVOID-in-Cosmetics-Skin-Care-Products-Infographic.html http://www.organicbeautytalk.com/ingredients-to-avoid/ http://www.davidsuzuki.org/issues/health/science/toxics/dirty-dozen-cosmetic-chemicals/ http://www.huffingtonpost.com/vanessa-cunningham/dangerous-beauty-products_b_4168587.html

2. **BHA (butylated hydroxyanisole) & BHT (butylated hydroxytoluene):** Found in lipsticks and moisturizers. Interferes with hormones, is a known allergen and is found to cause cancer in animals.

3. **DEA (diethanolamine), MEA (Monoethanolamine) & TEA (triethanolamine):** Found in moisturizers, shampoo and shaving cream. Banned in Europe because it is a known carcinogen.

4. **PEG (Polyethylene Glycol):** Found in many cosmetic creams. PEG is usually contaminated with the known carcinogen dioxane. Can also increase appearance of aging and reduce resistance to fighting bacteria.

5. **PG (Propylene Glycol) and Butylene Glycol:** Found in deodorants. The EPA requires workers to use protective gloves, clothing and goggles when handling PG — it is highly toxic, that's why it is used to take barnacles off boats. It is known to cause brain, liver and kidney abnormalities.

6. **Triclosan:** Found in toothpaste, antibacterial soaps, and deodorants. Classified as a pesticide, it is a suspected carcinogen, hormone disruptor and circulatory system suppressant.

7. **SLS (Sodium Lauryl Sulfate) & SLES (Sodium Laureth Sulfate):** Found in engine degressers, garage floor cleaners and 90% of personal care and cleaning products that foam. They are skin, lung and eye irritants. Can cause kidney and respiratory damage when combined with other common ingredients.

8. **Synthetic Fragrances:** Found in perfume, cologne, shampoo, bodywash and moisturizers. These unknown chemical compounds have been associated with allergies, respiratory issues and reproductive dysfunction.

9. **Phthalates:** Found in nail polish, perfumes, lotions, deodorants and hair spray. They are endocrine disruptors with links to decreased sperm counts, birth defects, and liver/kidney issues.

10. **Formaldehyde:** Found in nail polish, shampoos, conditioners, moisturizers and bodywash. It is a known carcinogen.

11. **Sunscreen Chemicals:** Common names are benzophenone, PABA, avobenzone, homosalate and ethoxycinnmate. These are endocrine disruptors that can lead to cancer, cellular malfunction and DNA damage.

Recipes for Natural Self-Care Products
– recipes by Katy Cox[14]

All Natural Homemade Shampoo Recipe

½ cup distilled water

¼ cup Dr Bonner's mild Baby liquid soap

2 tsp avocado or Almond Oil http://amzn.to/1VnGiNb

1/8 tsp Peppermint or Rosemary essential oil

1/8 tsp tea tree essential oil

10 – 15 drops of essential oils of your choice for scent (Lemon, Rose, Ylang ylang etc)

Put the above ingredients in a bottle (you could even reuse an old shampoo bottle). Shake well before each use.

Natural Conditioner

1 large Aloe vera leaf

2-4 drops Rosemary essential oil

Peel Aloe leaf and scrape out the clear Jell. Place in a liquidizer or small smoothie machine (bullet etc) and blend until no lumps remain pour into a small bottle and add the essential oil, shake well. After shampooing, remove excess moisture from hair and then massage in aloe gel. Allow the hair to absorb the treatment overnight or for at least an hour. No need to rinse, just brush through.

---

14 http://www.everessencenutrition.com

Probiotic Deodorant

1 tbsp. cocoa butter

1 tbsp. coconut oil

1 tbsp. shea butter

1 tbsp. beeswax

2 1/2 tbsp. arrowroot powder

1 tbsp. baking soda

1/4 tsp.vitamin E or Almond Oil

15 drops essential oils of your choice

2 contents of 2 probiotics capsules (look for strains that do not need refrigeration)

Aloe Vera Face and Body Wash

Use a small bottle or jar:

Add 1.5 oz (45 ml) aloe vera gel to the bottle

Add ½ oz (15 ml) avocado oil

Add 4 drops Frankincense essential oil (Boswellia carterii)

Close the bottle and shake gently

Shelf life is about a month

Natural Fluoride Free Toothpaste

Store in a small glass jar:

¼ cup baking soda

¼ cup coconut oil

1-2tsp fine Sea salt

5-7 drops essential oil (Thieves, Peppermint, cinnamon, clove, Tea Tree)

1tsp stevia powder or 4 drops liquid stevia (optional)

1-2tsp bentonite clay

1 capsule Activated charcoal (optional)

Blend dry ingredients, add melted coconut oil and essential oils, mix well and transfer into jar

Rich Body Butter

½ cup cacao butter

½ cup shea butter

½ cup coconut oil

6-8 drops essential oil or blend of oils

Gently heat all ingredients, adding the cocoa butter first, then shea then coconut.

Allow to cool in a mixing bowl and then add in your essential oils. Once the mixture has cooled transfer into a jar or pour into silicone moulds for cute 1 use portions.

Natural Makeup Remover

1 jar Coconut oil

Removes all makeup, dirt and impurities from the skin gently and with no disruption to the natural pH.

Allies in Body Beauty

There are many companies that are now making safe skin care products. One great way of finding high quality and safe products is from a local craftsman. You can also make them yourself — it is actually quite easy and fun.

If you have a smartphone, download the *Healthy Living* application and use it when you make your purchases. This application was designed by the Environmental Working Group to assist you in your quest for ultimate health. All you have to do is scan the product's barcode and the *Healthy Living* database will inform you if the product is safe or not. Another useful application is the *ThinkDirty*, which works similarly to the *Healthy Living*.

Here are also two suggested companies that I personally use for my body cleaning and sun protection products:

1. Simply Divine Botanicals: http://www.simplydivinebotanicals.
com
2. Badger Sunscreen:[15] can be purchased at most organic food or
health food stores.

Concepts for Food Cleansing

Brief Overview for Food Cleansing Attitudes

1. **What to Eat** The approach that we take for a food cleanse is
by eliminating wheat, dairy, animal protein, sugar and caffeine.
Fresh vegetables and low glycemic fruits will provide for a highly
alkaline diet, which promotes digestion, enzyme uptake, cellular
repair and weight loss. Include as many fresh vegetable juices and
smoothies as possible. (See the recipe section for healthy cleanse
appropriate recipes.) Eat as close to raw, organic and seasonal
vegetables as possible. Limit your consumption by using small
plates, taking breaks in between bites and enjoying the company of
others.

2. **Duration** Challenge yourself to try this approach for 5 days.
You can also make cleanse appropriate meals for one day or even
an entire month. One day liquid fasts are highly recommended
as well.

3. **Elimination** Cleansing does not have to be a full-on experience.
Consider eliminating one or two things from the "Avoid" foods
for a month or indefinitely. Just eliminate soda or coffee. Trying
going a week without wheat or fried foods and see how you feel.
Do a 10 day sugar cleanse and see how you feel.

4. **Addition** Bring in some of the "Alternatives" or "Enjoy" foods.
Try these foods for at least 1 month to allow your body to adjust.
When Gandhi would incorporate new food into his diet he would
try them for at least a month to see how they assimilated.

---

15   For other safe sunscreens visit, http://www.ewg.org/2014sunscreen/best-sunscreens/
best-beach-sport-sunscreens/

5. **Reverse Elimination** Shivanter Singh, healthy lifestyle strategist, suggests that when we re-introduce foods we do so with great mindfulness. Notice how that piece of cheese, cup of coffee or dessert makes you feel. This is a great way to build awareness around how your intake is actually affecting you.

Fasting

Fasting is another great way of cleansing the body. It is a practice that is a part of almost every major spiritual tradition — but you don't have to be spiritual to do one. One day, three day and week long juice or water fasts are quite beneficial for your physical organism. After day three the body's digestion turns itself off and all its energy goes to repairing itself, cleaning the blood, eliminating toxins and recharging its organs. Water fasts and juice fasts are common in many detoxification regiments as well as spiritual traditions. If you want to attempt a fast, please consult a professional because it is important to have guidance when first starting out.

Below are fasting guidelines suggested by Dr. Gabriel Cousens (excerpt from his book *Spiritual Nutrition*):

- Take an enema at least once per day. Some clinics recommend as many as three separate enemas per day. Colonics during the fast are excellent as well.
- Brush the skin for 3-5 minutes once or twice daily and follow this with a bath and skin scrub to remove the excess dead cells and draw more toxins out of the system.
- Get plenty of sunshine and do deep breathing exercises to help detoxify the skin and lungs.
- Get moderate exercise during the fast to help activate the system to eliminate toxins. This may include 30-60 minute walk, swim, sacred dance, and/or 16 minutes per day on a rebounder
- Practice daily Yoga for moving the lympathics, as well as general exercise

- Take short saunas to enhance perspiration, which helps the detoxification process
- Abstain from sexual activity to conserve energies for healing and regenerating.
- Use flower essences and gem elixirs during the fast to help balance and align the subtle bodies and chakras to awaken the chakras
- Scrap the tongue each day to remove toxins.

Chapter 6

Meditation

You should sit in meditation for 20 minutes a day,
unless you're too busy. Then you should sit for an hour.
—Zen saying

Many of us have preconceived notions about meditation: what it is, how we are supposed to "do it," what the effects are supposed to be and even what we are supposed to look like — I can assure you, it is not what you 'think.' If we review an average day we can find moments where we meditate already, where we enter the zone or a trance. Sometimes, time and thought seem to cease; and we become suspended, somewhere else. Other times we may "daydream" or visualize things in our mind's eye. Both thinking and not thinking are valuable types of meditation.

Meditation is a general term used for any type of mental practice that typically involves focus and concentration. Many of the most well-known teachers, leaders, artists and thinkers have advocated a meditation practice as a key component to their mental acuity and sharpness. They recognize that the mind can either be our greatest ally or our most challenging enemy. Eastern traditions like Buddhism, Taoism and Hinduism teach us to harness meditation so that it can be used as a tool to manage life's fluctuations. In Western models, like Christianity, silence is revered: Be still, and know that I am God. Psalm 46:10. Quakers honor silence and time for reflection as important for fine-tuning the mind's capabilities.

Let us cherish the concept of Noble Silence as something that can be useful, refreshing and powerful. It is not just another task that we have to do because we "think" we need it for balancing. Finding five to ten minutes a few times a day to stop, slow down and allow for our thoughts to drain has been shown to improve work productivity, communication, and emotional balance. The benefits are numerous and profound.

For many years I wanted to meditate; but I made excuses not to... When I did find time, I felt inadequate. I was also overwhelmed by the churning thoughts and unable to "quiet the mind." I felt like a failure and quickly gave up. Since, I have lessened my expectations and opened space for my thoughts. With a changed perspective on meditation, I no longer feel the need to do it "perfectly," whatever that means. I have now re-found the power of meditation and am inspired to calmly sit in silence several times a day. Because of meditation, I often gain insight into questions that I previously found to be challenging. And of course, rest, relaxation and greater fluidity in my day-to-day life have followed with continued practice.

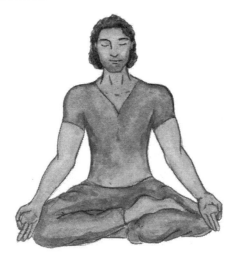

There are many types and styles of meditation filled with particularities and subtleties — so, how do we know where to start? Below are several types of meditations that are accessible, fun and effective. Try one or all of the techniques for at least one week and see what happens. Clearing the mind and maximizing its potential is not necessarily easy, but like anything else, a little practice goes a long way.

Unwinding the Day

The meditation technique of unwinding the day comes from Stuart Wilde's book *Infinite Self*. It encapsulates two of the key concepts of meditation: focus and concentration (with the intention of leading toward self-awareness). It is a great meditation on its own or can be used as a preparation for deeper meditative practices. The excerpt below describes the method:

> I've also taken time out each day to review the day. This process comes from the Hindu tradition and is usually done at night. It involves reviewing the day's events, in the mind's eye, running backwards through the day from bedtime to dawn. Don't ponder or comment too much on what happened — just watch. This exercise is a way of unraveling those experiences. It cuts down on the need for lots of trivial dreams, where the mind processes things that happened during the day. It's like moving backwards in time; it's a discipline to do just as you fall asleep so that you notice your life. Life will not be just passing you by; you're taking time to notice it. In reviewing the day's events, it unclutters the mind and allows you to go to sleep in a very pure state of consciousness. (Wilde 94).[1]

Notice the thoughts that take you out of this meditation. Become aware of how your mind can sidetrack itself. It is ok if this happens. Tangents are part of the process. They are the integration of an earlier experience. Witnessing yourself in the storyline and then assimilating it is the unwinding of static mental and emotional patterning.

---

1   This is only one of the many useful techniques that Wilde offers for personal and spiritual development. (*Infinite Self* is highly recommended to further your pursuit of Robust Vitality.)

Tratak

Tratak is another great meditation for cultivating focus and concentration. Enhancing focus and concentration can provide huge benefits when actively using our minds. Tratak is used to avoid mental distractions, improve mental clarity and memory, and refresh all aspects of overall consciousness. It is known to increase work efficiency and effectiveness, build confidence, strengthen will power and enhance quality of life. According to Matthew, Jesus once said: The light of the body is the eye: if therefore thine eye be single, thy whole body shall be full of light (Matthew 6:22). Could a practice like Tratak meditation be what Jesus was talking about? Fill the mind's eye with concentrated light and activate your inner luminosity.

TECHNIQUE

1. Light a candle and take a comfortable seat in front of it. It is best done with the candle at eye level in a still room. Sit 4 to 6 inches from the candle to start. Eventually, try it from different distances and see what happens.

2. When sitting, be comfortable and do your best to keep your spine straight. Sitting with poised grace and elegance is suggested. A soft, barely noticeable smile on your face enhances this practice as well.

3. Fix your gaze upon the candle flame with eyes open. Do your best not to blink. Tearing is great; but if you do not, that is ok. Couple this technique with deep breathing. On the inhalation, allow your stomach to expand. Allow the exhalation to be soft, easy and concentrated.

4. Imagine the flame entering into your body and illuminating your being. After approximately 7-10 minutes (if you cannot do 7-10 minutes at first, start with a time that is achievable and then work up to - minutes) allow your eyes to close. Bring the flame into your mind's eye, just as if you were seeing it with your eyes open.

5. [Optional] Bring in feelings of appreciation and gratitude and charge them with light. Bring in affirmations or other prayers and charge them with the light.[2]

6. Enjoy the effects.

7. Allow your eyes to open slowly.

Just as with other meditations, if thoughts arise, it is ok. Observe them and watch them pass by. This is a process of allowing the conscious mind to filter, file and integrate anything that you may be thinking. In time, you will become quite proficient at witnessing your thoughts or not experiencing them at all.

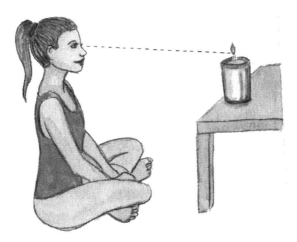

So Hum

So Hum is Sanskrit for "I am That." So = I am. Hum = That. "That" refers to all of creation. This is considered a mantra meditation. Remember, a mantra is word or phrase that is repeated with the intention of focusing the mind. Any mantra will work, but it is important to be mindful of the mantras that we are repeating. This is a traditional yogic meditation that is simple and great for beginners. The affirmative nature of the mantra is a great tool for bringing about peace and integration.

---

2 If you are familiar with the chakra concept, visualize the candle at each one to activate and purify.

TECHNIQUE
1. Take a comfortable seat with your spine straight. If you are sitting in a chair have your feet flat on the ground.
2. Breathe in and out through your nose and observe your breath without judgment or diagnosis.
3. On the inhalation say to yourself silently, "So."
4. On the exhalation repeat to yourself silently, "Hum."
5. If your mind begins to drift, bring your concentration back to your breath, then to your silent mantra.
6. Do this for 20 to 30 minutes.
7. Enjoy the effects.

Chapter 7

Self-Assessment and Personal Development Tools

Who looks outside, dreams. Who looks inside, awakes.
—Carl Jung

The cultivation of our conscious awareness can lead to the reality that we want. We can choose in almost all situations to be happy or sad. We can look at challenges as opportunities, mistakes as lessons and disturbances as a chance to grow. By starting with our thoughts, we can generate a positive attitude. "It isn't what you have or who you are or where you are or what you are doing that makes you happy or unhappy. It is what you think about it," Dale Carnegie, *How to Win Friends and Influence People*. In other words, our happiness depends on the quality of our thoughts. What is it that we are thinking about? How do we exercise our mind in a way to create a positive perspective?

In the information age, we are bombarded with ideas, thoughts, concepts, statistics and data. In my opinion, much of this information is opinion. We choose what we want to believe. Scientists have clued us into what is called the reticular activating system. It allows our brain to focus on the information it needs to accomplish a certain task and filter out what is not important.

Not only do we have to filter the "facts" that come to us directly, but we must challenge commonly accepted cultural beliefs, familial patterning and social influences. We are neither just a product of nature nor solely of nurture. By embracing both we are bound to neither. We are determined by the choices we make using our free will.

> Endowed with the ability to be self reflective, the self-conscious mind is extremely powerful. It can observe any programmed behavior we are engaged in, evaluate the behavior, and consciously decide to change the program. We can actively choose how to respond to most environmental signals and whether we even want to respond at all. The conscious mind's preprogrammed behaviors is the foundation of free will (Lipton 103).

What we do with what we receive (and what we give) is our choice.

Roger Bannister, the first person to break the 4-minute mile is a perfect example of this. Throughout track history the 4-minute mile was deemed impossible. In the 1940s, the mile record stood at 4:01. Scientists and publications declared that the human body could not move any faster and it was dangerous to even try [filter]. On May 6, 1954 Roger Bannister proved otherwise — he ran a mile in 3:59.4. Soon after, many runners broke through the previously thought impossible 4-minute mark — and today some high school athletes are able to accomplish this feat. How did he do it?

Part of his training was setting his mind to that task by visualizing the entire run [focus]. He exercised his muscle of awareness and prepared his body to accomplish the impossible. He created a mindset, which generated a specific state of being (vibration) for breaking the 4-minute mile. We are all beings of vibration and our resonance attracts "like" vibrations.

This "like attracts like," has become known as the Law of Attraction, made popular by the book *The Secret* and the film *What the Bleep Do We Know*. Quantum physicists use the term "quantum entanglement" to describe these interactions. One scientific example was discovered in

1665 when Dutch physicist Christiaan Huygens noticed his grandfather clock pendulums swinging in unison. They would sync up no matter when they were started.[3] This example can also be seen when groups of women get together for long periods of time and their menstrual cycles sync up. In the same manner, our thoughts — more importantly our feelings — generate the same sort of synchronizing vibrations. When in groups of likeminded and hearted individuals, these vibrations become intensely amplified.

Kareem Rosser, Daymar Rosser and Brandon Rease are a testament to the power of group energy. These young men were part of a program called Work to Ride in Philadelphia. They came from some of the worst neighborhoods in the city where some of their friends and fellow workers had been shot, killed, consumed by drug and/or gang violence or had chosen street life [filter]. Instead of street life, these boys chose to work in the horse stables in exchange for riding lessons. On March 13, 2011 they became the first all black team to win the High School Polo National Championship and are now rated some of the top polo players in the world [focus]. They, like Bannister, fixed their mind and practice on a goal and accomplished it, stunning the world.

Was it nature or nurture for them? What choices did they make that determined the trajectory of their lives? Where did they get their resilience?

Another incredibly true story of resilience is depicted in Lauren Hillenbrand's book *Unbroken*. It tells the tale of Louis Zamperini, a man with an unbreakable spirit. A former Olympic athlete in the 1936 games and WWII veteran survived nearly impossible conditions because he kept his mind sharp and heart inspired. After their plane was shot down, Zamperini and a fellow airmen survived over 40 days adrift on a raft in the Pacific Ocean, surrounded by sharks, with no food or water. He was then able to survive almost 3 years in the torturous Japanese internment camps [filter]. He and his comrades told each other stories and quizzed themselves daily in order to survive their horrid situation [focus].

---

3   http://www.nature.com/news/2002/020221/full/news020218-16.html

He was eventually rescued and returned to the United States with a severe case of post-traumatic stress syndrome. Again, he overcame the trauma by forcing himself to think and feel in new ways about his human experience. He went on to work as a motivational speaker until he died at age 97. He continually accomplished astonishing feats by maintaining an unwavering, positive attitude and productive mindset. We too have this capability.

This process begins with the quality of our thoughts. How do we remain unwavering in a turbulent world? What does it mean to have peace of mind? Awareness, practice and a little help from our friends goes a long way. If we have a burning desire for something and allow nothing to get in our way, then our mind/body will sync with the exact information that will get us there and disregard the rest (reticular activation).

Our mind is a very powerful tool that we must learn to use wisely. Buddhists have shown that it can also be a detriment, what they call "the drunken monkey." By focusing our attention, our consciousness, our mind on something, we become powerful transmitters of what it is, whether we want it or not. It might not be running a sub 4-minute mile, winning polo championships or surviving a torturous war, but these examples clearly state that anything is possible.

The following techniques can help shape your mind and heart to create the reality that you want.

The Magic of Thinking Big

In his book *The Magic of Thinking Big*, David J. Schwartz, Ph.D. discusses the importance of making goals and outlining a flexible plan. The Chinese proverb, "a journey of one thousand miles starts with a single step," presupposes that we know where we are going. We might not know how to get there, but we do know where we want to end up. In Chapter 12, "Use Goals to Help you Grow," he writes, "A goal is an objective, a purpose. A goal is more than a dream; it's a dream being acted upon. A goal is more than a hazy, "Oh, I wish I could." A goal is a clear "This is what I'm working toward" (Schwartz 159).

Schwartz, like many other great teachers of manifestation, suggests that we formulate an idea of what we want to accomplish — an intention for our life's purpose. The plan must be flexible to allow for the universe and all its co-conspirators to sync up with us. First we must set a goal. "Nothing happens, no forward steps are taken until a goal is established. Without goals, individuals just wander through life. They stumble along, never knowing where they are going, so they never get anywhere" (Schwartz 159). By setting our eye on the prize, we can allow for creative solutions to help us reach that goal. In short, "before you start out, know where you want to go" (Schwartz 160).

Schwartz suggests the following methodology with professional careers in mind; but it can be applied to things other than just work or finances. One of my teachers offers us a similar technique called "casting your seeds into the future." The practice was developed for massage sessions. He envisions how the client will feel after the session. This allows for his consciousness to partner with the client's (and with a greater, universal consciousness) to co-create that vision. This technique is easily adapted to other things like business sales, choosing a partner or earning a degree.

By creating goals and writing them down we offer prayers to the universe for the sake of the things we want. If we do not tell Santa Claus what to get us for Christmas, how is he going to know what to bring? What are you asking for?

Below is the Schwartz outline for a plan. Answer the following questions and notice your emotional connection to each one.

30 Day Improvement Guide (Schwartz 168-169)

Between now and _____, I will

A. *Break these habits:* (suggestions)

    1. Putting off things.

    2. Negative Language.

    3. Watching TV more than 60 minutes per day.

    4. Gossip.

B. *Acquire these habits:* (suggestions)
1. A rigid morning examination of my appearance.
2. Plan each day's work the night before.
3. Compliment people at every possible opportunity.

C. *Increase my value to my employer in these ways:* (suggestions)
1. Do a better job of developing my subordinates.
2. Learn more about my company, what it does and the customers it serves.
3. Make three specific suggestions to help my company become more efficient.

D. *Increase my value to my home in these ways:* (suggestions)
1. Show more appreciation for the little things my wife does which I've been taking for granted.
2. Once each week, do something special with my whole family.
3. Give one hour each day of my undivided attention to my family.

E. *Sharpen my mind in these ways:* (suggestions)
1. Invest two hours each week reading professional magazines in my field.
2. Read one self-help book.
3. Make four new friends.
4. Spend 30 minutes daily in quiet, undisturbed thinking.

10 Years' Planning Guide (Schwartz 161)

A. *Work Departments:* 10 years from now:
1. What Income level do I want to attain?
2. What level of responsibility do I seek?
3. How much authority do I want to command?
4. What prestige do I expect to gain from my work?

B. *Home Department:* 10 years from now:
1. What kind of standard of living do I want to provide for my family and myself?
2. What kind of house do I want to live in?
3. What kind of vacations do I want to take?

4. What financial support do I want to give my children in their early adult years?

C. *Social Department:* 10 years from now:

1. What kind of friends do I want to have?
2. What social groups do I want to join?
3. What community leadership positions would I like to hold?
4. What worthwhile causes do I want to champion?

Creative Workshop Process

The Creative Workshop Process, from the book *Ask and It is Given* by Esther and Jerry Hicks (155-161), is recommended to be done as a written exercise, but can also be done while driving, walking or during relaxation time. This process is used to awaken dormant energy — the "why" we want to do something. It begins to activate the energy in areas that we want to improve. It is also aimed at softening any resistance toward our goals. Focusing on the "why" rather than the "when" or "how" helps to harness an inner strength and conversely dissipate any resistance we may have toward accomplishing these goals.

The exercise requires us to take four pieces of paper and write the categories: My body, My Home, My Relationships, My Work. Write one on the top of each page. Write 3-4 statements of desire for each category. Each statement will be constructed with "I want..." sentences.

Example

MY BODY:

I want to feel fit and strong.

I want to live a long and fulfilling life.

I want to live pain free.

I want to have more energy.

Next, write 3-4 reasons under each statement of desire. The reasons should explain why you want the things you do. Use "...because..." statements to formulate these statements. Write 3-4 "...because..." statements.

Example

MY WORK:

I want to make more money...

> ... because I want to put my kids through college.

> ... because I want to go on an extra vacation this year.

> ... because I want to buy a new juicer.

> ... because I want to have a relaxing retirement.

Get creative with this exercise and enjoy the benefits. The intention of this exercise is to focus our energy on the *feeling states* that our desires will offer. When we source these *feeling states*, we will begin to attract the things we desire into our daily lives.

Personal Truth and Personal False

The *Personal Truth and Personal False* exercise is used for deprogramming our consciousness from destructive cultural programming. We have been conditioned throughout our lives with a lot of information and some of this information, this "stuff," can be detrimental to our overall wellbeing. Friends and family, marketers and advertisers, even doctors and legal advocates have been programming (consciously and unconsciously) thoughts, concepts and opinions into our psyches. These messages, mantras, ideas can become very powerful when repeated over time. By becoming aware of our self-talk, we can enhance our inner conversation.

So, what mantras are already embedded internally? What mantras do we want to repeat? This technique[4] was taught to me by Mukti, Michael Buck (founder of the Vedic Conservatory), with 3 powerful inquiries.

1. My most negative thought about myself is that I am...?

2. What am I afraid others will discover about me is that I am...?

3. I can't have the things the way I want them is because I am...?

Consider these questions heartfully. What do your instincts tell you right away? Record and ponder your answers to find out what may

---

4 He attributes learning this technique from his teacher Sondra Ray.

be lurking inside. Once you have settled on your answers, you then have a better understanding of the background mantras you have been telling yourself. Locate the one answer that has the strongest trigger, this is your personal false statement. It has a corresponding personal truth statement — what is it? Your personal truth will appear as the opposite pole.

Example

Personal False: I am not worthy
Personal Truth: I am worthy. I am valuable.

Personal False: I am not good enough.
Personal Truth: I am good enough.

Personal False: I am disingenuous.
Personal Truth: I am authentic.

To enter a new level of self-appreciation this is a very useful practice. For a mental refresher, repeat it as often as you want. Enjoy and celebrate your newfound awareness.

Chapter 8

Affirmations

Little by little, one travels far.
—J. R. R. Tolkien

Affirmations are written, verbalized or silently repeated sayings or expressions that are directed at our self and the world around us. Each has a specific intent. In the yogic tradition, they are called mantras. Just like practicing an instrument to perform a song, repetition of certain words and phrases, over long periods of time, has an impact on our lives. Is the song of our self composed of melodic or chaotic scores? How much and how rigorous are we practicing?

Whether it is an anabolic (positive) or catabolic (nonpositive) expression, our words can become powerful creators and real-time manifestations. By becoming aware of what we are telling ourselves, we can correct or enhance our mantras. If we put down or find problems within ourselves, we can easily put them into words. The same is true for life-affirming expressions. Affirming, or repeating, a mantra is a practice that can still the mind and generate vibrations for whatever it is we desire. What are you affirming?

The practice is simple: write down an affirmation (or several) many times a day. Read it, say it out loud and write it down again and again. This will train the (other than) conscious mind to have powerful default sayings that help improve and uplift our lives. Life-affirming expressions will frame a daily background to thrust us into *robust vitality*.

Note: when writing them use first, second and third person followed by your name to reinforce what it is you are affirming.

Template and Examples

I, [Your Name], ...
You, [Your Name], ...
He/She, [Your Name], ...

Examples

I, Joe, am abundant.

You, Joe, are abundant.

He, Joe, is abundant.

I, Suzy, am worthy.

You, Suzy, are worthy.

She, Suzy, is worthy.

This gives you a three-dimensional view of yourself and encourages the extra-you forces to help usher in or sustain your affirmation.

Example Affirmations

Career/Work I will direct all my energy toward my life's goals; and I will persevere.

Organization I have all the talents and abilities to manage my life's tasks.

Daily Life I make my way through my life openly and confidently.

Patience I remain calm and collected, secure in the knowledge that everything comes in its own time.

Self-Care I do well for myself and pay attention to my needs.

Sleep It is my intention to rest well and to awaken refreshed. And if there is anything important for me to recall from my dream state, I will recall it when I awaken (Hicks 195).

Spiritual I (say your name) see and draw to me, through divine love, those Beings who seek enlightenment through my process. The sharing will elevate both of us (Hicks xxiv).

Abundance I create prosperity easily and effortlessly. I love abundance and prosperity; and I attract it naturally.

Chakra Affirmations

First — Root Chakra belonging, safety, trust, connection to earth; I am safe physically and I belong here on earth. I have a right to be here.

Second — Sacral Chakra feelings, relationships, sexuality, creativity; I am a sensual and creative being. I have a right to feel pleasure in my body.

Third — Solar Plexus Chakra personal power, self control, vitality, purpose; I trust my own guidance and manifest my desires.

Fourth — Heart Chakra love, deep connection, forgiveness, compassion for self and others; I completely love myself and others.

Fifth — Throat Chakra communication, personal truth, expression, voice; I express myself clearly and in a healthy way.

Sixth — Third Eye Chakra intelligence, intuition, imagination, awareness; I have a sense of knowing everything I need to know.

Seventh — Crown Chakra connection with higher, spirit, source, creation, God, the universe; I am (So Hum).

Chapter 9

Communication

*We have two ears and one mouth
so that we can listen twice as much as we speak.*
—Epictetus

Communication is the seedbed for thriving interdependent relationships, for building community and for establishing a platform for creativity and growth. To enhance our communication skills — with ourselves and others — we can practice relating in ways that are nonviolent, compassionate and truthful. By taking a closer look at the practice of communication, we can learn to say what we mean and mean what we say.

Communication begins by connecting with our self first. What am I telling myself? What am I thinking? What impact do my thoughts have on my life? How am I communicating with my body and my emotions? What are my communication habits?

As we move outward and interact with others, the inquiry expands. We are now co-creating, in a more direct way, by verbalizing our thoughts and feelings — we must learn to differentiate between the two. Our interactions become opportunities for personal growth, community

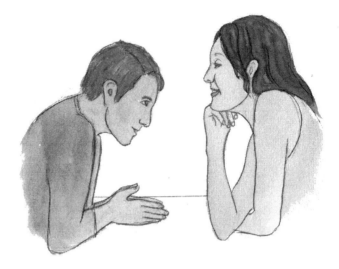

building and even global improvement. In these interactions, it is important to look at how we receive and respond to information. It is useful to ask: how am I presenting the information? How is that information being received? Are some forms of expression better than others? How can I refine my skills?

Communicative awareness first comes by observing our environment — what we see, exactly as it is. This is different than evaluating what we see. Notice if we are quick to judge, make assumptions, criticize or diagnose. Next notice what feelings arise from these stimuli. Are we happy, sad, stressed, uplifted, excited or...? How we interpret these feelings and express ourselves is a great opportunity for human connectedness. By practicing how we relate to each other, we can build meaningful and healthy relationships.

Oftentimes we speak without thinking. The lesson, "if you do not have something nice to say, do not say it at all," affords us a bit of space before we react to our stimuli. Remember, we are not just speaking with our words, tone, inflections; but we are speaking with our body and our emotions. We are not just communicating with other humans, but with plants, animals, the news, events, anything and everything in our world. Mindfulness practices for listening and speaking will be our focus for this section.

The Four Agreements
by Don Miguel Ruiz

The Four Agreements is an amazing book that offers wonderful guidelines for life. The four agreements are useful for almost any situation and give us a framework for interacting with people. This book is highly recommended. Below are *The Four Agreements* and a brief analysis of what Ruiz is offering.

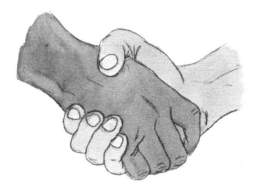

1. Don't Take Anything Personally

We are people with personalities, so how can we not take things personally? This is largely an exercise in nonjudgment and nonattachment. If someone becomes upset based on what you have offered, it most likely is not you. It is something from their past or a stored trauma; and though you may have been the trigger for their pain, you're not the cause of it. Not everyone knows how to connect with his/her emotions and express himself/herself in a compassionate way.

Compassionate understanding implies that we take into consideration things (about someone) that you might not know. Carry with you good intentions and whatever the outside world delivers is exactly what you need to learn and grow. The situation is usually bigger than what we think it is. We are in control of our actions and/or words, so notice the feelings that arise and take them as indicators for your own personal development. It is just another opportunity to evolve. By positioning ourselves in a place of nonattachment, we can communicate from a place of unconditional acceptance and respond with empathy.

2. Be Impeccable With Your Word

Many times we will say or commit to things without really thinking it through. The saying, "under promise and over deliver" is commonplace in the business world and with good purpose. Trying to accommodate for all the things you are asked to do can stretch you thin and cause undo stress. Take note of how your words and commitments are shaping your time, day and stress level. Offer what you can of yourself and if you offer too much, you will know by how you feel. Be cautious and judicious with your words and make good on your promises.

Being a person of integrity means holding true to your word. We must make realistic promises to people and fulfill them — in other words, no false advertising. Of course mistakes will happen, so own up to them and move on. Be honest, speak your truth, but remember the golden rule by *treating people the way you would want to be treated*. If you do not mean what you say, do not say it at all.

3. Don't Make Any Assumptions

Avoding assumptions helps us to limit our judgments and hard feelings towards others. This agreement brings up two other wonderful points of awareness: complaining and expectations. If we find ourselves complaining, we are most likely making assumptions about someone or something. The same goes for expectations. If we assume someone is going to do something, then we may set ourselves up for an unpleasant surprise if they do something differently. Reign in your expectations and be mindful of your complaints.

4. Always Do Your Best

This is something often directed at a little league baseball team or students in school. Whatever the outcome might be does not matter as long as you have done your best. You are the only one that knows if you have done your best, given your all or tried your "damnedest." You might not get what you want or what you think you deserve, "but if you try sometimes, you just might get what you need." This is another way of saying that with good intentions and a strong work ethic, you will receive exactly what you need in that space and time for growth and development. We might not believe it at the time; but it is a very useful philosophy during troubling times.

Similarly, recognize that everyone else is doing their best as well, whether they know it or not. It is a matter of inspiring them to dig and search a bit further — in a way that is compassionate — to find and access their greatest potential. Encourage others to do their best by doing yours.

Rotarian 4 Way Test

Herbert J.Taylor crafted the 4-way test in 1932 when he was asked to help revive the struggling Club Aluminum Company. He was a deeply religious man and prayed for a way to translate an ethical, nonpartisan, nonsectarian set of guidelines to help spur the company forward. He made several edits and checked with 4 department heads: a Roman Catholic, a Christian Scientist, an Orthodox Jew, and a Presbyterian. The department heads agreed that not only were they inline with their religious beliefs; but that they would be great for personal and business development. He designed these to be principles, rather than religious guidelines.

In 1942, Richard Vernor, director of the Rotary International, suggested it be used and in January 1943 the board ratified its use. Herbert J. Taylor became president of Rotary International in 1954-1955. Since then, it has been translated into more than 100 languages and helps to motivate direct, compassionate fulfilling dialogue. It is recited before every meeting.

4 Way Test for Everything You Think, Say or Do:

1. Is it the truth?
2. Is it fair to all concerned?
3. Will it build good will and better friendships?
4 Will it be beneficial to all concerned?

The Rotarian 4 way test and Ruiz's 4 agreements are useful concepts to carry with us. They give us a context for interacting with others. Review, reflect and apply them — see how your relationships change.

Kripalu Technique

The following technique is a powerful technique for communicating with someone on any topic, in a wide range of situations. By employing Kripalu Conscious Communication Technique, we can listen without judgment (as a "witness"), respond with empathy (allowing the other person to feel heard), and communicate our feelings and needs in a compassionate way. The content is taken from a pdf downloadable from the Kripalu website.

*Anywhere you see [], this indicates comments from the author of the manual.

Kripalu's Conscious Communication

Step One – Co-listening[1]

In co-listening, one person listens while the other person speaks. The listener practices listening without reply or response and with their full attention on the speaker. The listener practices non-judgmental awareness, "witness consciousness," for the speaker and self. There is no processing, interpreting, problem solving, analyzing, helping, or discussing during or after the co-listening process by either partner. The speaker notices what it is like to be listened to from someone listening from witness consciousness. When the designated time is up for the speaker the roles are reversed.

Step Two – Reflective listening

One person speaks while the other listens applying Co-listening. When the speaker is done (either a designated time has been set or the

---

1 Take a look at this website for more information on co-listening: http://www.dinaglouberman. com/approach/co-listening/

speaker finishes speaking), the listener repeats back to the speaker what they heard them say. The speaker then lets the listener know if there was anything they felt was not heard, acknowledged or was misheard. When this process is complete, the roles are reversed again.

Step Three – Conscious communication

This is a ten-step process. Covering each of these ten steps will ensure a complete communication. It is best for partners to apply Reflective Listening to these ten steps.

Setting the Stage

1. Is this a good time to talk? [Even though we may have something very important to share, it is appropriate to allow for the other person to be ready and willing to talk. This stage setting does not impose our will upon someone else who, for whatever reason, may not be ready to communicate.]

2. State intention to create harmony. [The word intention is used often and the difference between hard and soft intentions is necessary to grasp. A "hard" intention is something that we want to achieve. It is direct, clear, precise and more immovable than a soft intention. A "soft" intention is one that still focuses the conversation, but allows for something greater to take place. It allows for creativity, for a greater consciousness and for more than expected to happen. Try carrying soft intentions with you.]

3. Thank you for your willingness. [Sincere gratitude is very powerful. Use it often. Conscious communication, at any time, is a grateful celebration – so let us pay thanks.]

Whole Message

4. When you... (observable behavior — avoid statements of judgment)

5. I feel... (stay with feelings i.e. mad, glad, sad, bad, rather than judgments)

6. I imagine... (assumptions. Assume = ASS out of U and ME)

7. Which creates in me... (response)

8. I need... (state a primary need of yours i.e. "I need to feel respected," not what you need them to do for you.)

9. I ask... (state a request that is doable i.e. "I ask that you call me if you are going to be late.")

Closing

10. Thank you. [Notice this technique uses gratitude twice.]

After making a Conscious Communication, listen. Even if your partner is unaware of Kripalu Conscious Communication tools and may come from a defensive, attacking attitude. You can listen for the whole message including observable behavior, feelings, assumptions, reactions, needs and requests and be able to respond to them. This will help the speaker feel heard, understood, and perhaps help in working toward a quicker, smoother resolution. When Kripalu Conscious Communication is practiced often, it will become an authentic, communication and will not feel like you are using a "technique" on someone.

The 4 Components of *Nonviolent Communication*

In Marshall Rosenberg's Ph.D. book, *Nonviolent Communication*, he shares very powerful techniques for communicating in a way that is not only compassionate, but also gives us the tools for accessing deeper truths within ourselves. The following techniques are the essence of Rosenberg's work.

The art of nonviolent communication has 4 components:

1 Make observations.

2. Express how you feel.

3. Express needs from these feelings.

4. Make a request to fulfill your desired needs.

Notice the similarities between Rosenberg and the Kripalu Communication technique. Let us take a closer look.

1. Make Observations

Separate observations from evaluations. Really look at and observe what you see, not what you think you are seeing. By observing we enter into witness consciousness — "a place of nonattachment and unconditional acceptance." This enables us to parse out what we are witnessing, and what we are feeling about what it is we are seeing.

Start small and observe your surroundings: colors, shapes and sizes, etc. Say to yourself what you see, e.g. "revolving ceiling fan" or "floor ties." Not "spinning too fast" ceiling fan, or "dirty" floor tiles. For some people, the fan might be spinning just right or the tiles do not need attention. "The speed of the fan is making me cold," is a more accurate statement. "I noticed dirt on the tiles and since I like dirt less tiles, I'm going to clean them," is an observation and value statement. Try this simple practice of raw observation and see how it can reveal the difference between observations and evaluations. It might seem boring or even easy, but the practice heightens our sense of curiosity for what it is we are experiencing. It allows us to plant one foot firmly into the consciousness of the witness.

Take note of the thought patterns and words you are choosing when observing something. Are you observing or are you evaluating, i.e. judging, criticizing, comparing? Evaluations can bring us farther away from what we are observing, but can clue us into our internal landscape. "Analyses of others are actually expressions of our own needs and values" (Rosenberg 16). What are your needs and values? The answers lie in your internal and external dialogues.

If we make evaluative statements, it is not wrong or bad. We can use the things we say to our self and others as indicators of what is actually going on inside us. By probing our evaluations,[2] we see that there are two main types: 1) value judgments and 2) moralistic judgments. "Value judgments reflect our beliefs of how life can best be served. We make moralistic judgments of people and behaviors that fail to support

---

2 "Evaluations = judgments, criticisms, diagnoses, and interpretations of others are all alienated expressions of our own needs and values" (Rosenberg 61).

our value judgments, i.e. someone is good or bad because they are not honest" (Rosenberg 17).

Simply take note of what you are saying. This awareness will create that shift in consciousness that Eckhart Tolle writes about in his book *The New Earth* (see the introduction).

2. Express How You Feel

Distinguishing between thoughts and feelings can be quite helpful when communicating in a compassionate way. Sometimes it is not easy to verbalize how we feel. The more precise we get with how we feel the easier it is to work through (or with) that energy. Some helpful tips:

A. In general, feelings are not clearly being expressed when the word feel is followed by the words:

> that,
>
> like,
>
> as if pronouns
>
> names or nouns referring to people

Cultivate a mindful awareness around this concept and notice how we might misuse the word feel.

B. Work on building a vocabulary for feelings. *iGrok* or *Nonviolent Communication* are applications for the smartphone that can help with building this vocabulary.

Here are some words that express how we are interpreting others, NOT how we are feeling:[3]

> abandoned, abused, attacked, betrayed, bullied, cheated, coerced, cornered, distrusted, intimidated, let down, manipulated, neglected, overworked, pressure, provoked, put down, rejected, taken for granted, unappreciated, unseen, unsupported, unwanted, used.

Here are words that express feelings when our needs are being met:

> absorbed, affectionate, alert, alive, amazed, appreciative, blissful, breathless, calm, cheerful, comfortable, composed confident,

---

3   (Rosenberg 43-46)

curious, dazzled, delighted, elated, enchanted, encouraged, enthu-siastic, excited, expansive, fascinated, free, fulfilled, glad, grateful, happy, hopeful, inspired, interested, intrigued, invigorated, joyful, jubilant, loving, mellow, merry, optimistic, peaceful, pleasant, proud, radiant, refreshed, relaxed, satisfied, sensitive, serene, stimulated, tender, touched, tranquil, upbeat, warm, wonderful

Here are words that express how we feel when our needs are not being met:

afraid, agitated, alarmed, angry, annoyed, anxious, apprehen-sive, ashamed, beat, bitter, blah, bored, brokenhearted, cold, confused, cross, dejected, depressed, detached, disappointed, discouraged, disenchanted, disgruntled, disgusted, displeased, disturbed, edgy, embarrassed, exhausted, fearful, frightened, frustrated, furious, gloomy, heavy, helpless, hesitant, hostile, hot, hurt, impatient, irate, irked, irritated, jealous, keyed-up, lazy, listless, lonely, mad, miserable, morose, nervous, numb, overwhelmed, panicky, perplexed, puzzled, reluctant, repelled, resentful, restless, sad, scared, sensitive, shocked, sorrowful, surprised, terrified, troubled, uncomfortable, uneasy, unglued, unhappy, upset, vexed, withdrawn, worried

C. Go slowly. Breathe and allow yourself a moment to find the word that matches your particular emotion. I feel _____(emotion)_____ ...

3. Express Needs Based On Feelings

Once we have figured out our feelings, we can then express them and from there what "we are needing." A great technique for doing this is using the phrase "I feel... because I need..."

EXAMPLE:

I feel angry that she broke her promise, because I was counting on that extra time off from work.

I feel frustrated with spelling mistakes because I want my writing to be accurate.

I feel tired because I had a long day at work and I need some rest.

"The more directly we can connect our feelings to our own needs, the easier it is for others to respond to us compassionately" (Rosenberg 53). By being in touch with our feelings, then expressing our needs clearly, it makes it easy for others to satisfy those needs. Understand that other people (or things) cannot always satisfy our needs and that by developing a sense of self-reliance, we can make empowered decisions to forge our own happiness. The solutions to our needs may come instantly or overtime, either way we have begun to open ourselves up to greater opportunity for success.

"When our consciousness is focused on what we need, we are naturally stimulated toward creative possibilities for how to get that need met. In contrast, the moralistic judgments we use when blaming ourselves tend to obscure such possibilities and to perpetuate a state of self-punishment" (Rosenberg 133).

4. Make a Request to Fulfill Your Desired Needs

Requests can be very powerful and freeing if stated in a positive manner. We must allow the receiver the freedom to say "no." By doing so they have a greater ability to offer an authentic "yes." Here are some useful tips for making requests:

A. Use positive language to make requests.[4] Instead of telling people what we don't want, tell them what we do want. Avoid using words like "don't," "no," or "not." Instead try saying "I want...," "please can you...," or "I would like..."

B. Ask for concrete actions.[5] Do not be vague with your wording. Even requests like "can you please clean up your room?" can be interpreted in many ways. "Please make your bed, fold your clothes and put them away?" This is a more direct and concrete. By clearly stating what needs to be done, our requests can be honored directly. By minimizing our margin of error, there is less chance for confusion and emotional

---

4 (Rosenberg 67)

5 (Rosenberg 69)

disturbance. "When we simply express feelings, it may not be clear what we need. — Requests may sound like commands when unaccompanied by the speaker's needs and feelings." (Rosenberg 73).

C. Ask for the receiver's feedback to make sure that the message sent was the message received. Simply ask: "can you say back to me what you have heard."

D. Making requests vs. demands:[6]

When making a request we often want to know:

What the listener is feeling.

What the listener is thinking.

Whether listener is willing to participate in a particular action.

Distinguishing between a request and a demand is very important. Request from the speaker shows empathy. By showing empathy we allow for another's feelings to be expressed and needs to be met. We grant the receiver the ability to say no — they have a choice. Having a choice validates personal sovereignty and freedom.

E. Words to be aware of when asking for something:

should be,

supposed,

deserve,

justified,

right to

Requests turn into demands with words like these. We can request something and look for a response without stating a demand, in fact we often expect some sort of response. "My belief is that, whenever we say something to another person, we are requesting something in return... The clearer we are about what we want, the more likely it is that we'll

---

6 Awareness for requests and demands: Observe what the speaker does if the request is not complied to. Does the person willfully comply with your response even if it is contrary to their request? Do they become angry, sad or defensive? If it is a demand then the speaker criticizes or judges (Rosenberg 79) "Classifying and judging people promotes violence. Comparisons are a form of judgment" (Rosenberg 18). If the person lays a guilt trip then we can look to see what needs aren't being met and help them through the process of discovering their needs and feelings (Rosenberg 80).

get it" (Rosenberg 74). By using the 4 components of *Nonviolent Communication* we can be clear and precise in asking for things.

Listening and Responding with Empathy

As Chinese philosopher Chuang-Tzu stated:

"The hearing that is only in the ears is one thing. The hearing of the understanding is another. But the hearing of the spirit is not limited to any one faculty, to the ear, or to the mind. Hence it demands the emptiness of all the faculties. And when the faculties are empty, then the whole being listens. There is then a direct grasp of what is right there before you that can never be heard with the ear or understood by the mind." (Rosenberg 91)

What Chuang-Tzu is talking about is witness consciousness. It is a complete multi-dimensional experience that presupposes the listener holds no prejudices, biases or preconceived notions about the speaker.

I first listened with empathy on the streets of New York City with a friend. We set up a "Free Advice" booth on the street and for several hours we were busy listening, sharing and questioning our fellow street goers. The technique that we had employed, unbeknownst to us, had much to do with empathetic listening.

Despite the name of our street experiment, "Free Advice," we were not actually giving advice. Advice is an offering of what we feel or think about something, whereas empathy is to focus on the other person's message. We asked questions, listened and encouraged the inquirer to find their own resolution. We employed "say back" techniques and were conscious of our posture, eye contact and body language. It took us a few hours for us to learn the basics but we managed to assist many people without actually offering any advice.

The Buddhist saying "Don't just do something, stand there," is the suggested metaphor for listening empathically.[7] Being patient and

---

7 Dag Hammarskjold, Secretary-General of the United Nations, once stated, "The more faithfully you listen to the voice within you, the better you will hear what is happening outside." Be conscious of your inner dialogue and much will be revealed.

allowing the speaker to lead the conversation can provide tremendous relief for someone in a time of need. Dr. Rosenberg suggests that "the key ingredient of empathy is presence: we are wholly, present with the other party and what they are experiencing" (Rosenberg 94). By being present for our self and others we can offer presents into the present moment.

So, how do we listen empathically?

We employ the 4 components of nonviolent communication. "No matter what others say, we only hear what they are 1) observing, 2) feeling, 3) needing and 4) requesting" (Rosenberg 94).

A key component is to listen to what people need rather than what they are thinking. This helps us sift through any extraneous information where we may get caught up. Paraphrasing is a great technique for listening empathically. It is suggested that this be done in the form of questions. Phrase the questions based on what others are observing, how they are feeling, their needs based on those feelings, and what they are requesting. If we are going to ask for information, first we express our own feelings and needs then move to our inquiry.

A. When to paraphrase:
- When messages are emotionally charged.
- When it contributes to greater compassion and understanding.
- To slow down and truly be an active listener.

B. How to reflect back:
- Tone of voice is important. When hearing our own words reflected back, it could be sensitive, so we must be mindful of tone and speed of our words.
- Our tone indicates that we are asking whether we have understood – not claiming that we have understood.
- Look for key words and reflect them back to the speaker.

If our paraphrasing is met with resistance, we must recommit and focus on listening for feelings and needs. This can be tough because often we become entangled in what is going on in the other person. "Behind all those messages we've allowed ourselves to be intimidated by are just individuals with unmet needs appealing to us to contribute to their well-being" (Rosenberg 99). In the back of our mind we must remember that difficult messages are opportunities for us to help enrich and enhance someone's life by allowing them to be heard. If we get frustrated with someone else, it is ok, to express the feelings and needs around that frustration. As Rosenberg says "We only feel dehumanized when we get trapped in derogatory images of other people or thoughts of wrongness about ourselves."

There are numerous benefits to listening with empathy. We allow the speaker to access deeper parts of themselves. We access our emotional sovereignty by not carrying the burden of others. It is fun because we can empower others on their own journey. How then can we sense when the speaker has received adequate empathy? What are the indicators? Two indicators are: 1) a noticeable relief in tension, 2) the flow of words comes to a halt.

Taking Responsibility and Emotional Liberation

Taking responsibility for ourselves, i.e. our actions, feelings and words, is a powerful display of personal sovereignty. When it comes to our feelings, taking responsibility can be difficult at times, but quite liberating if we choose our words appropriately. When we project the cause of our feelings onto the world or someone else we give it power. We then become at the affect of those people, things and events making us a passive participant in the world. In life, just like the wind, our journey may be calm and still or turbulent and strong. By taking responsibility we can become co-creators of our emotional reality and provide ourselves with the healing balm needed for emotional fulfillment.

Embracing our emotional sovereignty is tested when we offer or receive a negative message. We must remember that, "What others do may be the stimulus of our feelings, but not the cause" (Rosenberg 49). This enhances our ability to get to the heart of what it is that we are experiencing. Is it the other person or what we harbor inside that causes an emotional stir? As St. Augustine once said, "hate the sin and not the sinner." Although hate is a hot emotional state, he is accurate in placing disdain on the action, rather than the person. To take it one step further, we can look at others as stimulants for our emotional learning experience. How we feel when things do not go our way is quite telling — we need to be open to these in tense moments. Unfriendly or violent communication between individuals does not serve in promoting higher levels of consciousness.

According to Rosenberg (Chapter 5), there are 4 different options for dealing with negative messages:

1. Blame ourselves [Blaming ourselves can be a representation of taking things personally. Remember Ruiz's four agreements, "don't take things personally."]
2. Blame others [Whenever we point the finger, we always have three pointing back at ourselves.]
3. Sense our own feelings and needs [This process gets us in touch with our inner landscape.]
4. Sense others' feelings and needs [We see ourselves in others and have begun the process of empathy.]

Valuing our needs is important when it comes to valuing ourselves. If we do not value our needs and ourselves, how can we expect others to? Recognizing our feelings, then finding our needs based on our feelings can be a very empowering process. It can lift us from "emotional slavery" to "emotional liberation" (Rosenberg 57). Dr. Rosenberg discusses 3 stages for emotional liberation:

Stage 1: Emotional Slavery. We see ourselves responsible for others' feelings.

Stage 2: The Obnoxious Stage. We feel angry; we no longer want to be responsible for others' feelings.

Stage 3: Emotional liberation. We take responsibility for our intentions and actions. "We respond to the needs of others out of compassion, never out of fear, guilt, or shame" (Rosenberg 60)

As we walk in emotionally liberated shoes, we find an empowered sense of our individuality partly with the use of the word "I." (Lazarus 76) Use I-statements to express your wishes, and avoid critical You-statements,

EXAMPLE

I feel angry. vs. You made me angry.

I feel sad. vs. They make me sad.

I want to be fulfilled. vs. You need to please me.

People who routinely use I-statements tend to get along with others and are much happier.[8] This speaks to the notion of self-reliance and personal sovereignty. Keep asking yourself: how am I framing my insights?

"Should"

Nonviolent communication inculcates a deeper sense of connection with our self and others. By being mindful of our words, we can encourage clear and meaningful conversations. A common teaching practice for young children is to tell them to "use their words" when faced with confusion, challenges and emotions. Let us expand on this concept and encourage the idea to "choose your words."

Choose your words as a guide for more fruitful relationships. Choose your words as tools for assessing your consciousness. Choose your words for personal growth and development. According to Dr. Rosenberg, "We use NVC to evaluate ourselves in ways that engender growth rather than self-hatred" (Rosenberg 130). So let's do it.

One of the ways to engender growth is to look at our word choices. For a long time, I had an unhealthy relationship with the word "should." I used it haphazardly without regard for its meaning, its intention or its power. This is a strong word and is used frequently without regard to its meaning.

"In our language there is a word with enormous power to create shame and guilt. This violent word, which we commonly use to evaluate ourselves, is so deeply ingrained in our consciousness that many of us would have trouble imagining how to live without it. It is the word should, as in "I should have known better" or "I shouldn't have done that." Most of the time when we use this

---

8 (Lazarus 77)

word with ourselves, we resist learning, because should implies that there is no choice. Human beings, when hearing any kind of demand, tend to resist because it threatens our autonomy — our strong need for choice. We have this reaction to tyranny even when it's internal tyranny in the form of should" (Rosenberg 131).

So wonderfully put. Try not to "should" on yourself or others. In the same way, statements about things we "must" do or "have to" do can be equally perilous where choice is concerned. Choose your words carefully; so that actions can be birthed from a place of life-affirming bliss, rather than shackled by submission.

In the *60-Second Shrink 101 Strategies for Staying Sane in a Crazy World*, Arnold A. Lazarus, Ph.D. and Clifford N. Lazarus, Ph.D. refer to it as, "the tyranny of should: known as "categorical imperatives," shoulds, ought's, and musts create anger and guilt" (Lazarus 29). Creating anger and guilt can be avoided. We can create happiness and joy by being conscious of our word choice, however subtle it may be.

Lazarus and Lazarus offer one type of solution: "Try to catch yourself each time you lay a should, or must on someone. Change the should into a request or a preference... Change should, ought, must into "I wish" or "I'd prefer" and see what happens" (Lazarus 29).

Another technique for replacing our language is through translating "have to" expressions to "choose to" offerings. This can be done in general during conversations; or it can be done through a writing process.

Step 1: List all things on paper that you tell yourself you "have to" do. Things that are not fun. These are your chores that take away your choice. By noticing how long or short the list is can give you a good indicator of how much you are enjoying your time.

Step 2: Clearly acknowledge that you are doing them because you choose to. Put the words "I choose to..." in front of everything on the list.

Step 3: Get in touch with the intentions behind your choices. "I choose to... because I want..."

When we begin to understand the "why" in things, it can help us with the "how." "With every choice you make, be conscious of what need it serves" (Rosenberg 137). We do things for many different reasons, all of which are legitimate; some perhaps need to be revisited so we better understand ourselves.

Possible awarenesses that could stir our inner states of peace are motivations driven by:

1. Money.
2. Need for approval.
3. To escape punishment.
4. To avoid shame.
5. To avoid guilt.
6. To satisfy a sense of duty.

Are these healthy motivations for our choices? What are they indicating about ourselves and why we do things? Do we have the power to change just through our language? I believe that a simple shift in our language is all we need to catalyze growth and personal development. We can learn many things by choosing and witnessing our words.

Anger

Anger is OK. We are allowed to be angry, even enraged, heated, boiling, perturbed or put off. These feelings can be great teachers, indicators, or alerts if we allow them to be. When they arise, "because" of a person or thing, it is important to remember: "the first step to fully expressing anger in NVC is to divorce the other person from any responsibility for our anger" (Rosenberg 141). They are the stimulus not cause. What others do is never the cause of how we feel. We are not at the emotional mercy of the world around us. We are powerful co-creators that attract the experiences that drive personal growth and sometimes, anger can be a part of that experience.

So, what is anger? "Anger is a result of life-alienating thinking that is disconnected from needs" (Rosenberg 143). It usually is a bundle of thoughts, feelings, expectations and attachments. It may be difficult in the moment, but investigating what is really going on is important to access and satisfy unmet needs.

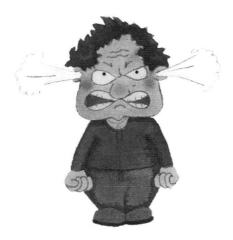

Anger can be an indicator of unmet needs, if we let it be. Allow it to be the "alarm" or opportunity clock for uncovering unmet needs. Switch the conversation from "I am angry because they..." to "I am angry because I..." When we become aware of our needs, anger (and many other emotions) dissipate and our creative impulses to fulfill those needs arise.

4 Steps to Expressing Anger

1. Stop. Breathe. [This tip can be applied to almost any area of conversation or expression. Tough personal questions, fearful or anxious situations, or confronting someone are all situations where breath is important. "Stop and breathe" is a great mantra for daily life.]

2. Identify judgmental thoughts. "The cause of anger is located in our own thinking" (Rosenburg 143). [Our mind can be a great friend or foe, it just depends how we use it. The thoughts that stir us to anger are useful clues that can be used to enhance our connection to our self or they can cause damage to our self and others. Our awareness of this gives us a choice on how to use these thoughts.]

3. Connect with needs. [Sometimes connecting with our needs is not easy; but by practicing it, we can become adept at finding our needs and feeling fulfilled just by knowing them.]

4. Express feelings and unmet needs. [By expressing feelings and unmet needs, we take the opportunity to be clear and concise without the

story or emotional baggage that is often accompanied with anger. Be mindful that when expressing feelings and unmet needs, the listener may not be able to fulfill our needs nor is it their responsibility. I had the need to be recognized by a former employer and realized that I, myself, must fulfill the need. This was a huge step in working on forgiveness, choice and personal sovereignty. As diligent as we may be about working on behalf of bettering ourselves, we must remember that not everyone is in a similar space — and that is ok. Validating our own self worth can be one of the most important lessons to learn.]

Chapter 10

Journaling Activities

True, This! -
Beneath the rule of men entirely great,
The pen is mightier than the sword. Behold
The arch-enchanters wand! - itself a nothing! –
But taking sorcery from the master-hand
To paralyse the Caesars, and to strike
The loud earth breathless! –
Take away the sword -
States can be saved without it![1] [2]

Our pen can act as a sword for slashing through old emotional chords, protecting our self from our self and for manifesting our wildest

---

1   Edward Bulwer-Lytton Richelieu; Or the Conspiracy, 1839

2   BulwerLytton may have coined the phrase but he was preceded by several others who expressed essentially the same idea: George Whetstone, in Heptameron of Civil Discourses, 1582, wrote, "The dashe of a Pen, is more greevous than the counterbuse of a Launce." In Hamlet, 1602, Shakespeare gave Rosencrantz the line "... many wearing rapiers are afraid of goose-quills and dare scarce come thither." Robert Burton's The Anatomy of Melancholy, 1621 includes "From this it is clear how much more cruel the pen may be than the sword." Thomas Jefferson sent a letter to Thomas Paine in 1796, in which he wrote: "Go on doing with your pen what in other times was done with the sword."

dreams. The Buddha was once quoted as saying, "the man who conquers himself is greater than one who conquers a thousand men on the battle field." Let our pages be our battlefield and the pen be our sword.

Journaling is a very powerful technique and can deliver huge results if we practice it. Many of our great leaders, like Abraham Lincoln and Martin Luther King, Jr. were avid note takers (along with being voracious readers and list makers). They always had pen and paper and were diligent about recording their experiences for the sake of enhancing their life and the lives of others. Even if you would not call yourself a writer, try journaling and see what happens. The sheer act of writing is enough to trigger thousands of biomechanical responses that elevate our vibration.

This section has all the questions from the previous sections under their specific heading. There are other questions under the heading "Contemplations" and "New Year's Reflections" to explore as well. When inspired, go through the list of questions and journal even if you only have a few minutes.

Contemplations

1. What question are you most afraid to ask?
2. Who in your life needs to be forgiven?
3. How can you have a vision so big that others want to be a part of it?
4. What am I grateful for?
5. What simple things can I do to change?

6. What are the 3 most important actions I can take to feel great on a daily basis?

7. How do I perceive time?

8. How do I view the world?

9. What are my biggest regrets?

10. What are my grandest dreams?

11. What do I want out of life?

12. Are you satisfied with the things you have? With your relationships? With your emotional and psychological landscape?

13. How do we get what we want on all levels? Where do we start? What do we do?

Space

Consider the feeling of your home

1. Is it inviting?

2. Are you happy to be in it?

3. Are the walls the color you want? Could you imagine something preferable?

4. Is the furniture the right size?

5. What sort of feeling does it provide for you when you think about it?

Imagine your office (studio, classroom, field, or wherever your workplace)

1. How does it help shape your life's purpose?

2. Does it inspire creativity?

3. Is it a place that attracts abundance?

4. Does it have a feeling of a second home or sanctuary?

5. What are your wealth goals? Is this the sort of place that you want to achieve them?

Mental/Emotional Clearing. Our minds are like a garden and we must tend to them with some regularity. Planting, watering and weeding are all parts of this process.

1. What needs to be planted?
2. What needs to be watered?
3. What needs to be pulled?
4. Which things are receiving love and which ones need more?

Physical Space

1. How does the design and placement of things impact your experience?

Self-Assessment

1. What are the quality of your thoughts?
2. How do you exercise your mind to create positive joyful brain-waves? 3. How do you remain unwavering in a turbulent world?
4. What does it mean to have peace of mind?
5. What mantras are you already telling yourself?
6. What mantras do you want to be hearing?

Breathing

1. How aware of your breath are you? How can you become more aware?
2. How does your breath change based on the situation you are in? Explain.
3. If someone asks you a tough question, how does your breath change? Explain.

Nutrition

1. What do you choose to eat and drink on a daily basis?
2. What types of snacks do you choose to eat? Keep a food journal for the week.

3. How do you feel right before you eat the food, during, 20 min. after, 2 hrs after?

4. What does health look like? Draw it, write it, mind map it.

5. What is health? Healthful? Healthy?

6. Have you ever explored notions of nutrition or contacted a specialist?

7. Have you ever considered body purification or detoxification or the notions of food as medicine?

8. Have you considered the environmental or political impact of your food choices? What about eating methods, i.e. chewing, saying prayers before or after, preparation, etc?

Purification

1. What are the steps to successfully complete a cleanse?

2. What are your intentions behind taking on such a practice? Why are you cleansing?

3. What does cleansing mean to you?

4. What is surfacing during the cleanse?

5. What am I resisting?

6. What is easy?

Affirmations

1. What scales are you playing to write the song of our self?

2. How much and how rigorous are you practicing?

3. What are you affirming?

Communication

1. What am I telling myself?

2. What am I thinking? What impact do my thoughts have on my life? How am I communicating with my body and my emotions?

3. What are the habits I have created around communication?

4. How am I presenting the information I have to offer to others and how is that information being received?
5. Are some forms of expression better than others?
6. Are you observing or are you evaluating, i.e. judging, criticizing, comparing?
7. What are your needs and values?
8. Take note of the thought patterns and the words you choose when observing something. Are you observing or are you evaluating, i.e. judging, criticizing, comparing? "Analyses of others are actually expressions of our own needs and values" (Rosenberg 16). What are your needs and values? Are these healthy motivations for our choices? What is it indicating about our self and why we do things? Do we have the power to change just through our language?

New Years Reflections[3]

The Year Past
1. What were 3 happy moments or events for you this past year?
2. What were 2 accomplishments you feel proud of?
3. What were the 2 most challenging times or issues?
4. What insights did you gain and how did you grow spiritually from these challenges?
5 What was the most significant blessing of the past year?

Coming Year
1. How do you want to live?
2. What changes do you want to make in order to live a happier, healthier, more meaningful, and freer life?
3. What's your intention for the coming year?
4. Write your mission statement for the New Year.
5. What do you want to accomplish in the New Year?

---

3   Grace, gratitude and many blessings to Todd Norian for offering us these questions and reflections.

6. What are two aspects of your life from the past year that worked well that you want to bring with you into the New Year?

7. What are 2 things you want to do differently in the New Year?

8. What's one habit or way of being that you want to let go of?

9. What's your vision for how to love and support yourself with respect to the following: Spiritual Practice, Diet, Exercise, Relationships, Work, Play

10. If you could wave your magic wand and create anything you wanted in the New Year, how would you live your life? What would you create?

Chapter 11

Superfoods

*"The doctor of the future will no longer treat the human frame
with drugs, but rather will cure and prevent disease with nutrition."*
—Thomas Edison

Super foods are an essential component for attaining and sustaining *robust vitality*. Some health experts have begun classifying these foods in their own category. They are certain types of food that are supercharged with beneficial nutrition. They are the best preventative medicines on the planet. These truly are foods that heal — incorporate them into your nutritional lifestyle!

Acai

Acai is a purple berry native to the Amazon, specifically Northern Brasil. It is loaded with antioxidants, more than blueberries and most other fruits. The pulp is fibrous and good for digestion. In 2008, the *Journal of Agriculture and Food Chemistry* reported findings that extracts from the acai berry destroyed cancer cells in a lab (Agin 147-149).

Acai is a standard breakfast in Brasil and it is easily prepared by blending it with other fruits, vegetables and nondairy milk. It can be made into a smoothie or prepared traditionally as a cold porridge to be eaten with a spoon.

Bee Pollen

Paavo Airola, author of *Worldwide Secrets for Staying Young*, reported about famed Russian biologist and botanist Dr. Nicolai Tsitsin who had surveyed over 150 people who were 125 years or older. He said: "All of the 150 or more people past 125 years old in Russia, without exception, have stated their principal food has always been pollen and honey — mostly pollen" (*Conscious Eating* Cousens 660-661). That is reason enough to incorporate bee pollen and honey into your diet. "Airola claims that honey boosts calcium retention, increases red blood cell count for nutritional anemia's stemming from iron and copper deficiencies" (*Conscious Eating* Cousens 661). Honey and bee pollen, in particular, are beneficial for arthritis, colds, poor circulation, constipation, liver and kidney disorders, poor complexion and insomnia.

Bee pollen is 20% protein, which is 5 to 7 times more protein than eggs, meat or cheese. It is 15 % brain building oils and lecithin, has 63 minerals and most B, C and E vitamins and 5,000 enzymes and coenzymes. It is also very high in antioxidants (*Spiritual Nutrition* Cousens 374-375).

According to Dr. Mercola, bee pollen contains all the essential components of life. It is considered an energy and nutritive tonic in Chinese Medicine. According to researchers at the Institute of Apiculture, Taranov, Russia,

> Honeybee pollen is the richest source of vitamins found in Nature in a single food. Even if bee pollen had none of its other vital ingredients, its content of rutin[1] alone would justify taking at least a teaspoon daily, if for no other reason than strengthening the capillaries. Pollen is extremely rich in rutin and may have

---

1 Rutin is an antioxidant that helps reduce inflammation and strengthen blood vessels.

the highest content of any source, plus it provides a high content of the nucleics RNA [ribonucleic acid] and DNA [deoxyribo-nucleic acid].[2]

There are many other studies that show amazing benefits of bee pollen and its positive effects for fighting cancer.[3] We highly recommend making this a staple in your diet.

Bee pollen can be sprinkled on salads or added to smoothies.

Cacao

Cacao is rich in antioxidant flavonoids, high in magnesium and contains tryptophan. Flavonoids reduce inflammation and protect cells from damage. Cacao is the highest whole food source of magnesium, which also happens to be the most deficient mineral in the diet of modern cultures (more than 80% of population is deficient in magnesium (*Spiritual Nutrition* Cousens 437)). Magnesium relaxes muscles, improves peristalsis in the bowels and relaxes the heart and cardiovascular system. Tryptophan, an amino acid, helps the brain produce serotonin, the happy chemical. The 2004, the *Journal of the American College of Nutrition* found eating 1.5 oz of dark chocolate improved blood vessel function. The 2005 *American Journal of Clinical Nutrition* showed flavonoids in cacao help improved insulin resistance (Agin 135-136).

---

2   http://www.mercola.com/article/diet/bee_pollen.htm

3   Dr. William Robinson of the Bureau of Entomology, Agriculture Research Administration published an article entitled: "Delay in the Appearance of Palpable Mammary Tumors in C3H Mice Following the Ingestion of Pollenized Food," Journal of the National Cancer Institute in October 1948, which showed that mice engineered specifically to die from cancerous tumors were improved due to bee pollen and some never developed tumors. These findings are stunning. At the University of Vienna, Dr. Peter Hernuss and colleagues conducted a study of twenty-five women suffering from inoperable uterine cancer and showed benefits from consuming bee pollen. Because surgery was impossible, the women were treated with chemotherapy. The women given bee pollen with their food quickly exhibited a higher concentration of cancer-fighting immune-system cells, increased antibody production, and a markedly improved level of infection-fighting and oxygen carrying red blood cells (hemoglobin). These women suffered less from the side effects of chemotherapy as well. Bee pollen lessened the nausea that commonly accompanies the treatment and helped keep hair loss to a minimum. The women also slept better at night. The control group receiving a placebo did not experience comparable relief.

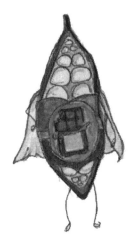

Dr. Gabriel Cousens conducted a study on the health benefits of chocolate in February of 2008. What he discovered was that raw cacao benefited diabetics as a safe food since it raises blood sugar less than almost any other food. It raises insulin sensitivity; and it is not toxic to the liver when combined in large amounts with sweeteners such as agave.

Some benefits of cacao include:

- It helps to activate phenethylamine, PEA, which is the feel good neurotransmitter responsible for the feeling of love!
- Encourages weight loss (because of its high chromium and coumarin content).
- Helps to prevent cavities (theobromine actually kills streptococci mutans one of the strains of bacteria that cause tooth decay).
- Regulates blood sugar which is beneficial for diabetes (chromium can naturally regulate blood sugar).
- Healthyeating.com sites *Journal of American College of Cardiology* and *The Journal of Internal Medicine* as having conducted respective studies which both showed decreased risk of stroke and heart attack with increased cacao intake.

Cacao powder can be used in smoothies. When combined with a banana and nondairy milk, it tastes delicious. The powder can also be used to make raw pudding by combining it with avocado and agave or honey. Try the nibs on there own for a bitter treat or combine them with dehydrated fruit like goji berries.

Chaga

Chaga is a fungus that grows on birch, alder, chestnut and hornbeam trees. It is an immune boosting agent that is popular in Europe and Russia. It has anti-inflammatory phenols, some of which demonstrate anti-tumor effects; hence its use in anti-cancer treatments. It also plays a beneficial role in metabolic disorders like obesity. The anti-oxidants found in chaga help to mitigate the effects of free radicals in the body.

It is best to cook the chaga in water. Gentle boil for 15-20 minutes and left covered to sit until the tea cools. Chaga can be consumed arm or cold. The grounds can saved and blended into smoothies.

Chia Seeds

Chia seeds are native to Mexico. The Aztecs and Mayans ate them before battle or making long treks for energy, endurance and to control appetites. Chia seeds contain large amounts of Omega-3 fatty-acids (more than flax), called alpha-linolenic acid (ALA), which is great for lowering cholesterol. Chia seeds are high in calcium, manganese and fiber and that carry a high percentage of protein. The 2007 *Journal of Diabetes Care* showed regular consumption of chia can lower blood pressure and reduce inflammation. Since they metabolize slowly, they help to regulate insulin and prevent hunger cravings, control blood sugar and boost energy. They absorb 7-10 times weight in water so soak them in water for at least 20 minutes before consuming (Agin 154-156). Chia pudding is a favorite of mine. Soak chia seeds for 20-30 minutes in water. Add cacao, goji berries, nondairy milk, coconut water, bee pollen and a touch of honey for a delicious superfood jump-start. It can also be added to juice and smoothies.

Chlorella

Chlorella is a fresh water algae which is good source of protein, fats, carbohydrates, fiber, chlorophyll, vitamins, minerals and "good" bacteria. It has a variety of curative effects including boosting the immune system, improving digestion, preventing colds, reducing cholesterol and hypertension, balancing pH and increasing energy levels. Chlorella is used for preventing cancer and mitigating radiation treatment side effects. Chlorella is also famous for its ability to bind to heavy metals, including mercury, and not bind with the metals your body naturally uses. It is essential for all detoxification regiments. Studies in Japan have shown that Chlorella may help reduce body fat percentage and in turn help with obesity and diabetes.[4]

Chlorella can be bought as tablets for oral consumption or in powder form to add to juices or smoothies. Chlorella's cell walls must be cracked for humans to be able to digest.

Coconut Oil[5]

Coconut oil is a great source of fatty acids. It can help prevent heart disease by lowering cholesterol. It protects hair against damage, can be used as sunscreen (blocks up to 20% of suns rays) and moisturizes the skin. It can boost brain function in Alzheimer's patients. Coconut oil is also useful in cleaning the mouth by pulling it through your teeth and swishing it around. It can prevent cavities and help to repair gums. Add it to smoothies, cook with it using low heat, use it as a carrier oil for essential oils, or spread it on toast.

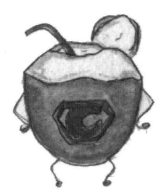

4   http://articles.mercola.com/sites/articles/archive/2012/02/01/is-this-one-of-natures-most-powerful-detoxification-tools.aspx#!

5   http://authoritynutrition.com/top-10-evidence-based-health-benefits-of-coconut-oil/

Flax Seeds

Flax seeds are high in Omega-3 fatty acids (ALA) and phytochemicals called lignins, which are antioxidants. They are high in fiber, B vitamins, magnesium, and manganese. It is the ALA that is good for the cardiovascular system and bones. Whole seed flax has soluble and insoluble fiber. Insoluble fiber dissolves in water and is good for regulating blood sugar and eliminating extra cholesterol. The *International Journal of Cancer* in 2005 showed lignins in flax inhibit growth of

Grinding is them best. It can then be added to salads, soups and smoothies. Flax oil is a great addition to meals as well. Dr. Max Gerson used flax seed oil as part of his legendary cancer treatment regiment.

Goji

Goji berries, also known as wolfberries, come from Tibet, China and the Himalayas. Goji berries are high in antioxidants and rich in vitamin A and C. They are high in antioxidants, beta-carotene and zeathanxin, which are special compounds that help boost immune function, protect vision and may help prevent heart disease.

Goji berries help fight cancer because of betaine. Betaine and beta-sitosterol lower cholesterol. The 1994 *Chinese Journal of Oncology* showed positive effects with cancer treatment. According to *Cellular and Molecular Neurobiology* March 2007, goji berries may have powerful effects for anti-aging because of the protection of nerve cells. These berries protect against age-related diseases such as Alzheimer's, dementia and Parkinson's. Other benefits include weight loss, heart protection and boost libido (Agin 156-158).

Goji berries are great as snacks. They can be included in trail mixes (great with cacao nibs), smoothies, cereal or oatmeal.

Hemp

Hemp is an excellent source of essential fatty acids as well as a complete protein source (*Rainbow Green* Cousens 149). Healthy fats help absorb glucose from the blood stream and turn it into energy, therefore good for diabetics.[6] Hemp is a source of Gamma Linolenic Acid (GLA), which is anti-inflammatory. This means it can reduce build-up of plaque in the arteries (which helps to improve circulation, lower cholesterol and lower blood pressure). The human brain contains many of the fatty acids found in hemp, which is good for prevention of Alzheimer's and Parkinson's. Hemp oil used on skin encourages new cell growth. It also contains all 10 essential amino acids (the building blocks of protein), magnesium, iron vitamin E, zinc, and phosphorus.[7]

It is great in soup, salad, smoothies, oatmeal and cereal; and the milk is delicious and a great alternative to cows milk.

Kombucha

Kombucha is a raw, fermented, probiotic, and naturally carbonated tea. It can improve digestion, fight candida (harmful yeast) overgrowth and produce alkalizing effects in the gut. It aids in the detoxification of liver and kidneys, which is useful for cleansing, preventing cancer and treating arthritis. As such, it is noted for reducing or eliminating the symptoms of fibromyalgia, depression, and anxiety.

It is extraordinarily rich in antioxidants, which boost immune system and energy levels. Try it, enjoy the bubbles and notice the effects.

Maca[8]

Maca is known as the "Peruvian Ginseng." It is a root vegetable grown at high altitudes. Maca stimulates hypothalamus and pituitary gland. These glands regulate adrenals, thyroid, pancreas, ovarian and testicular glands. In other words, it helps to balance hormones, which regulate and enhance such conditions as fertility, sexual function, digestion, brain and nervous system physiology, and energy levels. Maca is a

6 http://www.3fatchicks.com/7-health-benefits-of-hemp/

7 http://shine.yahoo.com/healthy-living/hemp-seeds-why-eating-superfood-171600844.html

8 http://macapowderbenefits.net

good source of B Vitamins, and has high levels of bioavailable calcium and magnesium. Maca works as an adaptogen, which means it responds differently to different people.[9]

Chris Kilham, author of *Hot Plants*, says, "Maca enjoys a very long history of successful medicinal use for menopausal discomfort, infertility and sexual healing. The question is not whether it works — because we know it works with certainty — but how it works."[10]

Maca is great in smoothies, oatmeal, and cereals.

Quinoa

Quinoa is a starchy seed native to the Andes and is considered an Old World grain. It is a complete source of protein, i.e. it contains all amino acids. It is also a source of magnesium, manganese, iron, copper and B vitamins. Quinoa is insoluble fiber, which is good for digestion, because it reduces risk of bloating, pain, and gas. The manganese and copper minerals help production of superoxide dismutase enzyme which helps fight off cell damage. The antioxidant activity helps to prevent cardiovascular disease, cancer and other inflammatory conditions. It helps migraines because magnesium relaxes blood vessels (Agin 126-128).

Try it as a substitute for rice or pasta. It can be eaten warm or in cold salads.

Reishi

Reishi is a mushroom that has been used for thousands of years to boost the immune system, reduce bodily stress, improve sleep and energize the body. It has been used in China and Japan in cancer treatment protocols for more than 30 years. In 2010, *Pharmacological Reports* published a study that showed ganodermic acid, found in reishi plays a role in inhibiting the development and metastasization of tumors.[11]

---

9   http://www.naturalnews.com/027797_maca_root_hormone_balance.html

10   http://www.webmd.com/sex-relationships/guide/the-truth-about-maca

11   http://www.sciencedirect.com/science/article/pii/S1734114010702528

In 2013, *Food and Chemical Toxicology* delivered a study that showed reishi mushrooms reversed chemical related liver damage.[12] In addition to aiding in liver repair and fighting cancer, reishi relieves for viral infections, high blood pressure, high cholesterol, kidney diseases, chronic fatigue, cardiovascular issues and general pain.

There is a reason they call this the "mushroom of immortality."

Spirulina

Spirulina is a microscopic blue-green algae. Spirulina is rich in gamma-linolenic acid (GLA), a compound found in breast milk that helps develop healthier babies. It has high levels of beta-carotene, which is good for healthy eyes, skin and anti-cancer protection. Spirulina has concentrated nutrient value, is packed with antioxidants, is easy to digest and promotes proper bowel functions. It has been proven to fight malnutrition in impoverished communities by helping the body absorb nutrients when no longer absorbs normal forms of food.

It acts as a natural cleanser by eliminating mercury and other toxins commonly found in the body. Spirulina increases stamina and immunity levels in athletes, and its high protein content helps build muscle.

Spirulina can be added to smoothies, green juice and soups. Now, we can even get pastas and chips made with spirulina.

Turmeric

Turmeric is an orange colored root native to India. It contains curcumin, which is a polyphenol, antioxidant and anti-inflammatory. It is commonly used in India as an Ayurvedic medicine. Turmeric regulates signaling mechanisms called cytokines, which helps to improve all functions of the body. According to the 2007 *Journal of Clinical Immunology*, curcumin is good for people with diabetes, arthritis, asthma, allergies and cancer. Turmeric is also found to have anti-cancer properties: *Biochemical*

---

12   https://www.mindbodygreen.com/0-15383/4-awesome-health-benefits-of-reishi-mushrooms.html

Pharmacology in 2007 showed that curcumin slowed growth of breast cancer. According to the *American Journal of Epidemiology* 2006, Asian women who ate curry with turmeric were less likely to get Alzheimer's than those that do not (Agin 145-146).

Turmeric is often dehydrated and ground into a powder. It can be used as a spice in addition to any meal. If you do not like the taste, pills are available. In root form, juice it, blend it into a smoothie or slice it and cook with it.

Wheatgrass

Wheatgrass is rich in vitamins A, B complex, C, K, iron and potassium. It is loaded with chlorophyll and is used to help detoxify and fight cancer. The 2002 *Scandinavian Journal of Gastroenterology* found that wheatgrass helped people with ulcerative colitis, an inflammatory disease of colon. It is an antibacterial that stimulates healing (Agin 162-164). Wheatgrass implants are common and used at the Hippocrates Institute for combating a variety of illnesses including cancer.

Drink it on its own, implant it, or mix it with juice.

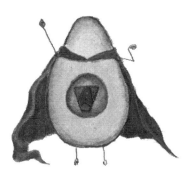

Chapter 12

Recipes for Healthy and Delicious Meals

One cannot think well, love well,
sleep well if one has not dined well.
—Virginia Woolf

Juices

Watermelon Mint

    2 cups cubed watermelon

    1 handful fresh mint

Green Apple, Carrot, Cucumber, Celery, Kale

    1 Green apple

    2 carrots

    1/2 - 1 cucumber

    4-6 stalks of celery

    6-8 leaves of kale

191

Honeydew, Cucumber, Cilantro, Lime
>1 cup honeydew
>1/2 cucumber
>handful cilantro
>1/2 lime

Liver Cleanser (Tico's Juice Bar, Princeton, NJ)
>1 Lemon with Peel
>1 Red Apple
>1 Carrot
>1/4 head Cabbage
>1 stalk Broccoli
>1/2 clove of garlic
>1/4 red onion
>handful parsley
>small bunch of mint
>small bunch cilantro

Bunny Brier's Patch (*Joe Cross 101 Juice Recipes*)
>1/2 yellow squash
>2 leaves kale
>1 apple
>1 stalk of broccoli
>2 handfuls spinach
>3 carrots

Cancun (*Joe Cross 101 Juice Recipes*)
>6 leaves of Kale
>1 cucumber
>1 lime
>1 small handful of mint
>1 jalapeno
>3 ribs of celery

Green Fennel Delight (*Joe Cross 101 Juice Recipes*)

    1 fennel

    1 rib celery

    8 leaves of kale

    1 green apple

    1 orange

Green Lemonade (*Joe Cross 101 Juice Recipes*)

    1 green apple

    2 handfuls of spinach

    8 leaves kale

    1/2 cucumber

    2 ribs celery

    1 lemon

    1" ginger

Summer Green (*Joe Cross 101 Juice Recipes*)

    2 pears

    4 leaves kale

    1 handful spinach

    1/2 cucumber

    1 zucchini

    1/4 lemon

    1" ginger

Gerson Juice Recipe (Dr. Max Gerson Recipe: www.gerson.org)

    1/4 to 1/2 of a dark green lettuces (depending on the size of the lettuce): red and green leaf lettuces, romaine, endives. (Iceberg is useless and do not use)

    2 or 3 leaves escarole

    2 to 3 beet tops (young inner leaves)

    5 or 6 leaves of Watercress

    2 or 3 leaves red cabbage

    1/4 green bell pepper

    a little Swiss chard

    1 green apple

Non Dairy Milk

Almond

> 1 Cup Soaked Almonds
>
> 2 ½ Cups Water
>
> 3 Dates (optional)
>
> ½ tsp vanilla extract (optional)

Soak almonds for 8 to 12 hours. Add 1 ½ cups of water, almonds, dates and vanilla into a blender and blend on high speed until smooth. Add the remaining cup of water and blend until smooth. Place a mesh strainer or cheese cloth over a bowl and strain. Press the pulp with a spatula to get out the remaining liquid. Compost the pulp or use for baking. Transfer the milk into a sealed container (preferably air tight, such as a mason jar) and keep in the refrigerator. Enjoy for up to 5 days. The milk will separate, so shake well before using.

Hemp

> 3 cups of water
>
> 1 cup of raw shelled hemp seeds
>
> pinch of salt
>
> 3 to 6 dates (optional)
>
> ½ - 1 tsp of vanilla extract (optional)

Put all ingredients into a blender and blend on high speed until smooth. Use the whole milk to maximize nutrition or strain using a strainer or cheese clothe. Compost the pulp if discarding. Transfer the milk into a sealed container (preferably air tight, such as a mason jar) and keep in the refrigerator. Enjoy for up to 3 days. The milk will separate, so shake well before using.

Oat

> 3-5 cups of water (depends on taste preference)
>
> 1 cup rolled or whole oats
>
> 1 tsp of vanilla extract (optional)
>
> 3-6 dates (optional)

Soak the oats for at least 20 minutes (overnight is preferable). Rinse and drain oats. Add all the ingredients into a blender and blend on high until smooth. Place a mesh strainer or cheese cloth over a bowl and strain. Press the pulp with a spatula to get out the remaining liquid. Compost the pulp or use for baking. Transfer the milk into a sealed container (preferably air tight, such as a mason jar) and keep in the refrigerator. Enjoy for up to 4-5 days. The milk will separate, so shake well before using.

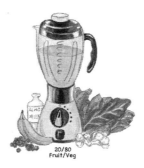

Smoothies

The Basic Chocolate

1 banana

2 dates

almond milk

coconut water

3 tsp. raw cacao

2-4 handfuls of spinach

The Super Chocolate

1 banana

2-4 leaves of kale

1 Tbsp. raw cacao

1 Tbsp. dehydrated goji berries

1 tsp. spirulina

1 Tbsp. chia

2 cups coconut water

The Spin-Appleini (chef Shivanter Singh)

    1/2 apple

    1/2 cup spinach

    1 celery stalk

    1 tsp. tahini

    1/2 banana

    2 cups water

The Ginger-Mint Green (*Liquid Raw* p. 33 from Dave Biddison)

    2 cups water

    2 whole apples, washed and chopped coarsely (seeds and all)

    2 cups fresh spinach, washed and packed

    1/2 lemon, juiced

    1 tsp. ginger, pureed

    10 leaves fresh mint (approximately)

The Pear-Mint Marvel (chef Shivanter Singh)

    4 pears

    4 leaves kale

    1/2 bunch mint

    2 cups water

Julian's Morning Delight

    1 banana

    2 Tbsp. chia seeds (soaked)

    1 date

    1 carrot

    3 leaves of romaine lettuce

    1/8 tsp. bee pollen

    1 cup coconut water

    1 cup almond, hemp, or coconut milk

The Popeye (*The Kid Friendly ADHD & Autism Cookbook* p. 124)

    2 cups baby spinach

    1/2 banana, ripe

1 cup water

4 to 6 ice cubes (about 4 ounces)

The Hemp Water Pear Power

1 pear

1/4 bunch watercress

2 tsp. hemp seeds

1/2 cucumber

coconut water

1/2 tsp. maca

hemp milk

The Un-Coffee

1 banana

2 tsp. raw cacao

3 tsp. coffee alternative (Roma, Pero, etc)

coconut water

3 pieces romaine lettuce

1 tsp. spirulina

nondairy milk

The Berry Delicious

handful blueberries

handful strawberries

handful raspberries

almond milk

1 tsp. of ground flax seed

2 tsp. ginger

1/2 lemon wedge

coconut water

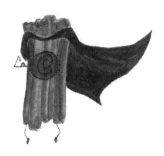

Breakfast

Hot Buckwheat, Banana, Flax and Walnuts (*The Ultra-Metabolism Cookbook* p. 162)

    Serves 4   Serving Size: 2/3 cup

    1 cup buckwheat groats, whole

    2 cups plain almond, hemp, soy, or coconut milk

    1/4 tsp. ground cinnamon

    pinch kosher salt

    1 small banana, mashed

    2 Tbsp. flaxseed, ground

    2 Tbsp. chopped walnuts

Place the buckwheat, milk, cinnamon, alt and mashed banana in a medium saucepan. Bring to a boil, stirring frequently. Cover the pan and reduce heat to low. Simmer for 15 to 20 minutes, until the buckwheat is tender. Top with ground flaxseeds and chopped walnuts

Applet-Walnut Amaranth (*The Ultra-Metabolism Cookbook* p. 163) Amaranth is a nutty, nutritious grain full of vitamins, minerals and protein.

    Serves 4   Serving Size: 2/3cup

    1 cup amaranth

    3 cups plain almond, hemp, soy, or coconut milk

    1/4 tsp. ground cinnamon

    pinch kosher salt

    1 large apple, skin on, cored or diced

    1/2 cup chopped walnuts

Place amaranth, milk, cinnamon, salt, and apple in a medium saucepan. Bring to a boil, stirring frequently. Cover pan and reduce heat to low. Simmer for 25 to 30 minutes until amaranth is soft. Top with chopped walnuts and serve.

Peach Quinoa with Flax and Nuts (*The Ultra-Metabolism Cookbook* p. 164) The South American grain, quinoa, along with flaxseed serves up plenty of protein and healthful omega-3 fats.

    Serves 4   Serving Size: 2/3 cup

    1 cup quinoa, thoroughly rinsed and drained

    2 cups plain almond, hemp, soy, or coconut milk

    1/4 tsp. ground allspice pinch kosher salt

    2 medium peaches, peeled, pitted, diced or 1½ cups frozen
        peaches

    2 Tbsp. flaxseed, ground

    2 Tbsp. chopped hazelnuts

Place quinoa, milk, allspice, salt, and peaches in a medium saucepan. Bring to a boil, stirring frequently. Cover pan and simmer on low heat for approximately 20 minutes, until quinoa is tender. Top with ground flaxseed and chopped hazelnuts.

Berry Breakfast Quinoa (*The Reboot with Joe Juice Diet* p. 138)

    Serving: 1

    1/2 cup quinoa

    1 cup water

    1/2 cup almond milk

    1/4 cup blue berries dash of sea salt

    Topping (optional)

    1 Tbsp. whole almonds

    1 Tbsp. hemp seeds

    dash of honey

1. Place the quinoa and water in a saucepan or rice cooker over a medium-high heat and bring to a boil, stirring occasionally.

2. When boiling, lower the heat, stir once, and simmer, uncovered for 10-12 minutes, until all the water is evaporated.

3. Add the almond milk, blueberries, and salt, and simmer for a further 3-5 minutes, stirring occasionally.
4. When the texture resembles porridge/oatmeal, serve with the topping of your choice.

Chia Cereal (chef Madeleine Ezanno)
2 cups soaked chia seeds
2 cups of almond milk (homemade almond milk 1 cup of almonds soaked over night with 2 cups of water strained through a nut bag. Can add a date to sweeten and a 1/4 tsp. of vanilla)
pinch of sea salt
1/2 Tbsp. sweetener (coconut nectar, honey, maple syrup or stevia)
1/4 tsp. vanilla or any extract such as almond, orange, chocolate (optional)
cinnamon with sliced apples
berries (of choice)
bananas
1. Soak the chia seeds for 2-4 hrs
2. Blend chia seeds slightly to give a creamy texture (can be stored in frig for 2-3 days)
3. Add other ingredients as desired

Autumn Morning Porridge (*Rainbow Green Live Food Cuisine* p. 371)
2 Cups butternut squash, peeled and cubed
1 Cup walnuts
1 Cup coconut water
2 vanilla beans
2 tsp. cinnamon
2 tsp. orange zest
Process all ingredients in a blender until smooth and creamy.

Apple Spice Porridge (*Rainbow Green Live Food Cuisine* p. 370)
2 1/2 cups coconut water
2 cups almonds, soaked
1 cup coconut pulp

> 1 cup apple, chopped
> 1 Tbsp. cinnamon
> 1 tsp. nutmeg
> 1 tsp. celtic sea salt

Process all ingredients in a blender until smooth and creamy. Serves 4-6.

Amaranth Porridge (*Conscious Eating* p. 687)

> 1 cup amaranth, sprouted
> 1/4 figs, soaked
> 1/2 cup fig soak water
> 1/2 ripe banana

Blend all the ingredients until smooth. In a pot, warm to 115 degrees F until hot to touch. Serve and enjoy.

Quinoa Pudding (*Conscious Eating* p. 688)

> 2 cups almond milk
> 1 cup quinoa, sprouted
> 1/4 cup almonds, sunflower seeds, or walnuts, soaked (and blanched)
> 1/4 cup raisins, soaked
> 1/2 tsp. cardamom
> 1/2 tsp. cinnamon
> 1/2 tsp. fennel
> 1/4 tsp. nutmeg
> 1/4 tsp. cloves
> Raw honey or raisin soak water to taste

Blend until smooth and serve.

Banana-Millet Porridge (*Conscious Eating* p. 688)

> 1 ripe banana
> 3 cups millet, sprouted
> 2 cups raisin or fig soaked water
> 1 tsp. cinnamon (optional)
> 1/4 tsp. nutmeg (optional)

Blend all ingredients until smooth

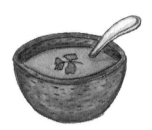

Soup

Bell Pepper Soup (*Liquid Raw* p. 78 from
Raw Chef Dan, Quintessence, New York, NY)

    3 cups filter water
    1/4 cup cold-pressed olive oil
    1 tsp. sea salt
    1 tsp. caraway seeds
    2 medium cloves garlic
    2 medium red or yellow bell peppers (discarding the green stems)
    2 medium cucumbers, chopped
    1/2 medium red onion, chopped

Blend ingredients in a high-speed blender until creamy and smooth.
Serve room temperature or chilled.

Creamy Mushroom Soup with Parsley Garnish (*Liquid Raw* p. 89 from
Sheryll Chavarria www.rawcanrollcafe.com)

    2 cups almond milk
    1/2 cup celery
    2 cups mushrooms
    1 Tbsp. tahini
    1 tsp. cold-pressed olive oil (optional)
    1/4 cup parsley or scallions, finely chopped (for garnish)
    1 Tbsp. white miso (or to taste)

Place all the ingredients into a high-speed blender and blend until lightly
creamy, being careful not to over-blend. Serve in bowls and garnish with
parsley or finely chopped scallions.

Watercress-Pear Soup (*Liquid Raw* p.104 from Potlucker Mary Kane)

  2 pears
  1/2 cup pecans, soaked (4 - 6 hrs.)
  2/3-1 Tbsp. allspice
  2 Tbsp. pumpkin seed oil
  1/2 bunch watercress
  1/4 cup cold-pressed olive oil
  1 cup filtered water
  Sea salt to taste

Blend all of the ingredients together in a high-speed blender to desired consistency. Some folks like this soup creamy and smooth, while others like the pear chunky and the watercress chopped so it is more visible. See what works best for you.

Green Detox Soup (*The Reboot with Joe Juice Diet* p. 129)

  Servings: 4
  2 garlic cloves
  1 leek
  small head of broccoli
  6 kales leaves
  1 zucchini
  2 celery sticks
  2 Tbsp. olive oil
  4 cups vegetable stock
  handful parsley, chopped
  sea salt and freshly ground pepper (to taste)

1. Chop garlic and all the veggies.
2. Warm the oil on low heat, then add the leek and garlic and cook slowly for 3-5 minutes.
3. Add the stock and the remaining vegetables and bring slowly to a boil. Cook for just a few minutes, until the zucchini is soft. The less you cook the vegetables the better.

4. Add salt and pepper to taste, then blend or process the soup to the desired consistency, from smooth to chunky.
5. Serve the soup in bowls and sprinkle with parsley.

Euphoria Soup (Golden Bridge Yogi's Cleanse Manual)
>   2 medium beets, trimmed
>   2 medium carrots, trimmed
>   1 large cucumber, skinned
>   1/2 cup avocado, mashed
>   1/3 cup cilantro leaves, loosely packed
>   3 cup filtered water
>   2 Tbsp. lemon juice
>   1 Tbsp. Braggs Liquid Aminos
>   1 clove garlic, crushed
>   1 small Serrano chile, stemmed, seeded
>   1 tsp. onion powder
>   1/2 tsp. cumin

Finely grate first 3 ingredients. Toss in large bowl. Place 3 cups grated veggies in blender, puree with all other ingredients until smooth. Pour puree into bowl of grated veggies. Stir & serve, or chill. Garnish with cilantro.

Vegetable Stew (*Conscious Eating* p. 700)
>   2 cups potatoes, chopped
>   3/4 cup cherry tomatoes, dehydrated
>   1/2 tsp. curry
>   1/8 tsp. cayenne
>   1 handful raw dulse, kelp, or alaria, soaked
>   4 cups water

Place all ingredients in a pot and heat at 115 degrees Fahrenheit until warm.

Upbeet Soup (*Conscious Eating* p. 705)
>   2 cups fresh carrot juice
>   1/2 cup beet, grated

1/2 cup carrot, grated

1 avocado

Blend ingredients until smooth. Garnish with sprouts.

Split Pea Soup (Golden Bridge Yogi's Cleanse Manual)

8 cups water

1 pound dried split peas (about 2 1/4 cups)

1 medium onion

2 cloves garlic, minced

1 tsp. dried thyme

1 tsp. salt pinch of cayenne pepper

2 to 3 carrots, chopped (on green days make without the carrots)

2 to 3 stalks celery, chopped

1. Rinse peas and pick out any stones, etc. Heat water and peas to boiling. Boil for 2 minutes, then remove from heat and cover. Let sit for 1 hour.

2. Add onion, garlic, thyme, salt and cayenne pepper. Cover and simmer until peas are tender, about 1 hour.

3. Stir carrots and celery into soup. Cover and simmer until veggies are tender, about 45 minutes.

Cucumber-Dill Soup (*Conscious Eating* p. 703)

1 large cucumber, chopped

1 red pepper, chopped

1 carrot, shredded

1 cup mushrooms, chopped

1 cup spinach, finely chopped

1 cup string beans

1/2 cup raw tahini

1/4 cup fresh parsley, minced

1 clove garlic

juice of 2 lemons

Celtic sea salt to taste

2 cups water

Blend water, tahini, lemon juice, and garlic. Combine with remaining ingredients and add Celtic salt to taste. Garnish with parsley.

Wild Sweet Corn Bisque (*Euphoric Organic Cuisine*)
>   Serves 2-4
>   2 cups think almond milk
>   1/2 cup almonds, soaked overnight (4-8 hours)
>   2 cups water
>   4 ears fresh corn (4 cups)
>   1 clove garlic
>   1 tsp. coriander seed, fresh ground
>   1/2 tsp. cumin seed, fresh ground
>   sundried sea salt to taste

1. Soak 1/2 cup almonds in 2 cups water (4-8 hrs) Drain and rinse almonds
2. Blend 2 cups fresh water and soaked almonds at high speed until smooth.
3. Pour blended almonds through strainer. Save pulp for other uses.
4. Saw fresh corn kernels from the cob.
5. Blend almond milk, corn, garlic, coriander and cumin seed in pulses until mixed but not smooth.
6. Season with sea salt to taste and set aside.

Salad

Ginger Lentil Sprout Salad (*Golden Bridge Yogi's Cleanse Manual*)
>   2 1/2 cup sprouted lentils
>   1/2 cup celery, finely chopped
>   1/2 red onion, minced (approx. 1/3 c)
>   1 Tbsp. ginger, fresh, minced
>   1 1/2 Tbsp. Braggs Liquid Aminos
>   1/2 Tbsp. olive oil
>   1 1/2 Tbsp. lemon juice 3
>   sheets nori, toasted and small pieces
>   1/4 cup soaked hiziki (seaweed)

Kale Salad (*Golden Bridge Yogi's Cleanse Manual*)

    2 large handfuls of kale, de-stemmed and chopped

    1 tomato

    1 small red onion, diced

    1 red pepper, thinly sliced

    Dressing:

    1/4 cup apple cider vinegar

    1/2 cup olive oil

    splash of lemon juice

    salt and pepper

Combine salad ingredients in bowl. Blend or whisk dressing until combined. Top with dressing and massaged salad with hands until reduced in size and wilted.

Greek Salad (*Conscious Eating* p.710)

    5 cucumbers, sliced

    5 tomatoes, diced

    1 cup olives, pitted and diced

    2 Tbsp. raw apple cider vinegar

    2 Tbsp. virgin olive oil (optional)

    1 Tbsp. oregano

    Celtic salt to taste

Radicchio Salad with Hazelnut Dressing (*Hungry for Health* p. 111)

    1/2 cup hazelnuts (filberts), chopped

    1/2 small head radicchio

    1/4 head Romaine lettuce

    6 Belgian endive leaves

    2 large white mushrooms, sliced

    2 Tbsp. lemon juice

    2 Tbsp. extra virgin olive oil

    1 Tbsp. maple syrup

Clean and shred all leafy vegetables. Toss with mushrooms and set aside. Combine lemon juice, oil, maple syrup and hazelnuts. Toss salad leaves with nut dressing until well coated.

Sunny Green Salad (*Conscious Eating* p. 711)

    1 avocado, sliced

    1 handful of kale, chopped

    1 handful sunflower sprouts

    1/3 cup sunflower seeds sprouted

Toss kale and sunflower sprouts with dressing. Decorate with avocado slices in a pinwheel design and top with sunflower seeds.

Farm Style Cabbage and Apple Slaw (Emily's Café) with shredded carrot and toasted sunflower seeds-dressed with agave mustard and poppy seed dressing.

    2 cups shredded green cabbage

    2 cups shredded red cabbage

    1 large green apple grated or thinly sliced

    1 large carrot, grated

    1/4 cup toasted sunflower seeds

    Dressing:

    1 clove garlic

    1/2 tsp. organic mustard

    juice of half a lemon

    1/2 cup olive oil

    2 Tbsp. raw agave

    2 Tbsp. poppy seeds

    dash of sea salt

1. Combine the cabbages, apple, and carrot in a medium mixing bowl.
2. Combine the garlic, mustard, lemon juice in a food processor and begin blending. Slowly add the olive oil and agave and continue blending. Season to taste with sea salt. Add poppy seeds.
3. Add the dressing to the cabbage and apple and mix well. Refrigerate before serving and mix well again. Add the sunflower seeds before serving.

Grains

Spiced Quinoa Millet (*Golden Bridge Yogi's Cleanse Manual*)

    1 cup millet

    1/2 cup of quinoa

    4 cups of water

    3 cloves garlic

    1/2 inch of ginger grated

    1 chopped onion

    1/2 tsp. of basil

    1/4 tsp. of parsley

    1/4 tsp. of oregano

    1 Tbsp. of Bragg Aminos

Place all the ingredients in a covered saucepan and simmer on low for 45 minutes or until the millet has absorbed the water.

Millet Tabouli (*Golden Bridge Yogi's Cleanse Manual*)

    3 cup cooked millet

    1 large cucumber

    1 bunch of green onions

    1 lg bunch of parsley

    1 stalk of celery

    1 sprig of mint

    1 Tbsp. fresh dill

    3 Tbsp. extra virgin olive oil

    1 ounce of fresh lemon juice.

    Optional: 1 clove or garlic or to taste

Refrigerate the cooked millet to cool it before using. Peel the cucumber, and fine chop the cucumber, green onions, parsley, celery, mint, garlic and dill. Mix the ingredients with olive oil and fresh lemon juice. If you like it wetter, you can add more olive oil and lemon juice.

Tabouleh, My Way (*Food Matters* p. 190)

    Serves: 4 1/2 cup fine-grind (#1) or medium-grind (#2) bulgur

    1/3 cup olive oil, or more as needed

1/2 cup freshly squeezed lemon juice, or to taste

1 tsp. salt and freshly ground black pepper

1 cup roughly chopped parsley leaves

1 cup roughly chopped mint leaves

1 cup peas or fava beans (frozen are fine, just run them under cold water to thaw)

6 or 7 radishes, chopped

1/2 cup scallions

2 medium tomatoes, chopped

About 6 black olives, pitted and chopped, or more to taste

1. Soak the bulgur in 1 1/4 cups boiling water to cover until tender, 10 to 20 minutes, depending on grind. If any water remains when the bulgur is done, put the bulgur in a fine strainer and press down on it, or squeeze it in a cloth. Toss the bulgur with the oil and lemon juice and sprinkle with salt and pepper. (You can make the bulgur up to a day in advance. Cover and refrigerate; bring to room temperature before proceeding).

2. Just before you're ready to eat, add the remaining ingredients and toss gently; taste, adjust the seasoning, adding more oil or lemon juice as needed, and serve.

Sweet and Spicy Creamy Coconut Corn "Chowder" Sauce — with steamed Quinoa and Veggies (Madeleine Ezanno)

2 cups of quinoa cooked

Creamy Coconut Corn Chowder Sauce

3 cups of fresh corn off the cob or frozen organic corn

1 1/2 to 2 cups of organic unsweetened coconut milk

1/4 cup of pine nuts (optional)

1 Tbsp. light miso

1-2 Tbsp. Olive oil

1 1/2 Tbsp. fresh squeezed lemon juice

half of a jalapeño chopped

1-2 tsp. of coconut nectar

1 tsp. coconut aminos

a handful of fresh parsley for garnish (or any fresh herb of choice)

1. Blend all ingredients in a high speed blender until smooth (I like to leave a handful of corn on side unblended)
2. Heat sauce in a pan, pour over steamed quinioa. Add cooked veggies of your choice, grilled, sautéed or lightly steamed.

Quinoa with Vegan Basil Pesto and Roasted Sweet Potato (Emily's Café, Pennington, NJ.)

> 1 3/4 cup water
> 1 cup organic quinoa
> 1 medium to large organic sweet potato
> 1/3 cup pine nuts (or walnuts, or both)
> 2 - 3 Tbsp. cold pressed organic extra virgin olive oil
> 5 cloves garlic
> 1/3 cup nutritional yeast
> 1 bunch fresh basil (or 3 cups of your favorite, seasonal herb, arugula, or broccoli rabe)
> sea salt and pepper to taste

1. Combine water and quinoa in a medium saucepan; bring to a boil. Cover, reduce heat, and simmer 20 minutes or until liquid is absorbed. Remove from heat; fluff with a fork.
2. Place the pine nuts in a skillet over medium heat, and cook, stirring constantly, until lightly toasted.
3. Gradually mix the pine nuts, olive oil, garlic, nutritional yeast, and basil in a food processor, and process until smooth. Season with salt and pepper.
4. Peel the sweet potato and dice into approximately 1/2 inch cubes. Coat with 3 Tbsp. olive oil and season with salt and pepper. Spread onto a baking sheet and roast in a 375 degree oven for approx. 20 minutes or until tender and slightly browned.
5. Combine the quinoa, pesto and sweet potatoes and enjoy!

Vegetable Dishes

Easy Lettuce Wraps (*The Kid Friendly ADHD & Autism Cookbook* p. 176)

   Servings: 4   Serving Size: 2 wraps

   8 whole Boston or Bibb Lettuce leaves, washed and dried

   2 cups filling of choice of chopped vegetables

   1/3 cup dressing

Tender lettuce leaves stand in for bread in these easy, quick roll-up sandwiches. This is a good way to be clever about including new kinds of vegetables (remember start with a small amount well mixed in with vegetable favorites). If diet is low in protein, this is a tasty way to include more.

Fill each lettuce leaf with 1/4 filling. Sprinkle with a couple tsp. of dressing and then roll up like a burrito.

Thai "Peanut" Sauce Vegetables (*Crazy Sexy Diet* p. 218 offered by Chad Sarno www.rawchef.com)

   Serves 4

   1/2 cup almond butter

   1 Tbsp. fresh ginger, chopped

   1 1/2 Tbsp. lemon juice

   2 cloves garlic

   1 1/2 Tbsp. sea salt

   1 tsp. Serrano pepper, diced (optional)

   1/3 cup water, plus more to thin sauce

   2 zucchini, sliced in half moons

   2 carrots, julienned

   1 cup broccoli florets

   1 cup snow peas

   1/2 cup cilantro, chopped

In high speed blender, blend the almond butter, ginger, lemon juice, garlic, salt, Serrano pepper, and water until smooth. Add water as needed to achieve desired thickness. Toss the sauce with vegetables and cilantro in large mixing bowl. When the vegetables are tossed well, dehydrate on Teflex sheets at 105 degrees F for 2-3 hours to soften.

Choosing Raw "Peanut" Noodles (*Crazy Sexy Diet* p. 219-220 contributed by Gena Hamshaw, www.choosingraw.com)

> Serves 1-2
>
> For the Asian Dressing (Makes 1 1/2 cups):
>
> 1" piece gingerroot
>
> 1 cup olive oil (or flax oil)
>
> 2 tsp. toasted sesame oil
>
> Juice of 1 lime
>
> 1/4 cup mellow white miso
>
> 6 dates, pitted, or 1/4 cup maple syrup
>
> 2 Tbsp. of nama shoyu
>
> 1/3 cup water

Blend all ingredients on high till creamy and emulsified.

For the Noodles: 1 large or 2 small zucchinis, spiralized or sliced with a vegetable peeler 1/2 red pepper, sliced into matchsticks 1/2 carrot, sliced into matchsticks 1/4 large or 1/2 small cucumber, grated or peeled into long strips scallions or green onions to garnish

To make dish, simply prepare and mix all vegetables, save the scallions or green onion. Toss them with 1/4 cup dressing, adding more if necessary, and sprinkle with scallions. Sugar snaps, shiitake mushrooms, snow pea shoots, or mung bean sprouts would also be a great addition to the noodles.

Not Your Usual Ratatouille (*Food Matters* p. 206)

> Makes: 4 to 6
>
> 1 medium or 2 small eggplants (about 8 ounces)
>
> salt
>
> 1/4 cup olive oil
>
> Freshly ground black pepper
>
> 1 small head cauliflower, trimmed and cut into florets
>
> 1 small onion, chopped
>
> 1 tablespoon minced garlic
>
> 1 red bell pepper, cored and chopped
>
> 2 medium tomatoes, cored and chopped

1 Tbsp. chopped fresh thyme

1/2 cup chopped basil leaves for garnish

apple cider vinegar or freshly squeezed lemon juice, optional

1. Trim the eggplant and cut it into large cubes. If the eggplant is big, soft, or especially seedy, sprinkle the cubes with salt, put them in a colander, and let them sit for at least 30 minutes, preferably 60. (This will help improve their flavor, but isn't necessary if you don't have time). Then rinse, drain and pat dry.

2. Put 2 tablespoons of the oil in a large skillet over medium heat. When hot, add the eggplant, sprinkle with salt and pepper, and cook, stirring occasionally, until soft and golden, about 10 minutes. Remove from the pan and drain on paper towels.

3. Put the remaining 2 tablespoons oil in the pan and add the cauliflower. Cook, stirring occasionally, until it loses its crunch, about 4 minutes. Add the onion, garlic, and red pepper and cook and stir for another minute or two, until they're soft. Add the tomato and thyme and cook for another minute, until the tomato starts to release its juice. Return the eggplant to the pan, along with basil leaves. Give a good stir, taste and adjust the seasoning, and serve hot or at room temperature, with vinegar or lemon. The ratatouille will keep for a couple of days, covered and refrigerated.

Parsnip Rice Avocado, Vegetarian Sushi — with a sweet and spicy ginger sauce (chef Madeleine Ezanno)

Parsnip Rice:

1/2 lb of parsnip

1/4 lb pine nuts

1. Shred the parsnips in a food processor

2. Change blades, pulse shredded parsnips adding the pine nuts until its rice like size

Ingredients: 4 sheets of raw or toasted sushi nori pea sprouts, alfalfa sprouts 4 romain leafs sliced very thinly 1 avocado sliced (squeeze lemon or lime juice to prevent browning) 2 carrots shredded 1/2 cup of chopped raw unsalted almond, pecans, or walnuts (optional) 1 cup of hot water to seal the nori

Dipping sauce: 1/4 cup of coconut amino 1/4 tsp. red chile pepper paste 1/4- 1/2 inch piece of ginger grated 1/4 tsp. of coconut nectar a few drops of toasted sesame oil 1/4 cup of coconut milk (optional) 1/4 cup of almond butter (optional)

1. Place nori sheet on a sushi rolling mat or clean dish towel onto a cutting board
2. Spread the parsnip rice mixture evenly across the bottom half of the nori sheet
3. Add 1/2 teaspoon of dipping sauce, avocado slices (about 2), carrots, sprinkle nuts, sprouts
4. Seal at the ends with warm water

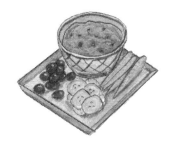

Dips and Sauces

Mexican Guacamole (*Karo's Nutritious & Delicious Cruelty-Free Dishes*)

   Serves: 4-6

   2 fully ripened Avocadoes diced

   1/4 cup minced onion, divided

   1 Tbsp. (or more to taste) jalapeno chiles divided

   3/4 tsp. sea salt

   1/2 cup finely chopped plum tomato

In a medium bowl, place 2 tablespoons of chopped onion, the chiles, and 1 tablespoon of the salt. Mash with the back of a wooden spoon, until the mixture becomes a juicy paste. Place avocados in the bowl with the paste; stir to combine. Fold in the tomato and the remaining onion.

Fresh Salsa Recipe (*Karo's Nutritious & Delicious Cruelty-Free Dishes*)
    2 bunches coriander, washed, dried, leaves and stems chopped
    2 ripe tomatoes, finely chopped
    1 small red onion, finely chopped
    4 fresh red birdseye chiles, halved, deseeded, finely chopped
    1 large garlic clove, finely chopped
    1/4 cup olive oil
    2 Tbsp. fresh lemon juice, or to taste
    salt and ground black pepper, to taste

Place coriander, tomatoes, onion, chilles, garlic, oil, lemon juice, salt and pepper in a medium bowl. Stir well to combine. Taste and add more lemon juice, salt or pepper, if necessary. I personally find that salsa tastes the nicest if you refrigerate it for a few hours before serving.

Raw Mint Beet Dip (chef Madeleine Ezanno)
    2-3 beets cleaned and peeled
    1 Tbsp. chickpea miso (or light miso)
    1/4 lemon juice squeezed
    handful of mint or any fresh herb, parsley, dill, cilantro
    1/4 cup of pine nuts, raw unsalted pecans or almonds

Blend in a food processor until smooth, drizzle organic cold pressed olive oil as needed to help blend.

Artichoke Dip (chef Madeleine Ezanno)
    1 jar of artichoke hearts in water drained
    1-2 cloves of garlic
    1/4 lemon juiced
    1/4 tsp. of light miso or 1/2 Tbls of nutritional yeast handful basil
    1/4 cup cold pressed organic olive oil
    1/4 cup nuts (optional)

Blend in food processor until smooth (guacamole texture).

Non Dairy Pesto (chef Madeleine Ezanno)
    Serves: 4-6
    1/4 cup of raw unsalted pecans, walnuts

1 bunch of basil 1 Tbsp. nutritional yeast
1/4 cup of cold pressed organic olive oil

Italian Broccoli Dressing (*Kripalu Kitchen* p. 134)

Yield: 5 cups
6 cups cooked broccoli
Tomato Sauce:
3/8 cup tomato paste
1 1/2 cups water
1/8 cup lemon juice
1/2 Tbsp. tamaric
1 tsp. basil
1 tsp. dill
1/2 tsp. black pepper
1/4 cup oil

Cook the broccoli thoroughly; drain and allow it to cool. While the broccoli is cooking, you can prepare the tomato sauce by mixing the tomato paste and water or by using already prepared sauce. Add the broccoli, sauce and remaining ingredients, making sure to blend well so that the dressing has a creamy consistency.

Dressings

Hemp Seed Dressing (*Rainbow Green* p. 258)

1 tomato
1 small carrot
1/2 bell pepper
1/8 cup hemp oil
1/2 Tbsp. lemon juice
1/2 tsp. Celtic Salt

In a blender, process all ingredients until smooth and creamy. Makes 1 1/2 cups.

Red Pepper Curry Dressing (*Rainbow Green* p. 263)

> 1 cup red bell pepper, chopped
>
> 1/4 cup olive oil
>
> 2 Tbsp. lemon juice
>
> 1 Tbsp. curry powder
>
> 1/2 tsp. Celtic salt

In a blender, process all ingredients until smooth and creamy. Makes 1 1/4 cups.

Caesar Dressing (*Rainbow Green* p. 254)

> 3 avocados
>
> 1/3 cup lemon juice
>
> 1 Tbsp. black pepper
>
> 1 Tbsp. salt 1 tsp. cayenne
>
> 3 Tbsp. olive oil
>
> 1/4 cup water

Blend all ingredients together in a high-powered blender. Makes 2 cups.

Creamy Cuke Dressing (*Rainbow Green* p. 255)

> 1 large cucumber
>
> 1/3 Cup flax oil
>
> 1 Tbsp. raw tahini
>
> 2 tsp. dill
>
> 1/2 Tbsp. Celtic salt

In a blender, process all ingredients until smooth and creamy. Makes 1/2 cup.

Hot Mustard and Poppy Seed Dressing (adapted from *Conscious Eating* p. 717)

> 2 cups mustard seeds, soaked
>
> 1 cup raw apple cider vinegar
>
> 1 tsp. Celtic sea salt
>
> 1/4 cup lemon or lime juice
>
> 1 Tbsp. poppy seeds
>
> 1/4 cup water, add more water, if needed

Blend all ingredients until smooth.

Cucumber, Lemon and Dill Dressing (*Kripalu Kitchen* p. 126) Yield: 3 cups

    2 cups cucumbers
    1 cup lemon juice
    2 Tbsp. honey
    3 Tbsp. oil
    1 tsp. kelp
    1 Tbsp. dill weed
    3/4 cup sunflower seeds

Chop the cucumbers, making sure all the outer skins are first peeled off, and add them to the blender along with the other ingredients. Prior to adding the sunflower seeds, blend the mixture once so that it becomes liquid in consistency; then slowly add sunflower seeds, making sure these get thoroughly blended.

Parsley – Tahini Dressing (*Kripalu Kitchen* p. 129) Yield: 1 1/2 cup

    3/4 cup parsley
    1/2 cup tahini
    1 Tbsp. lemon juice
    1/2 cup water
    1 tsp. tamari dash cayenne

Chop the parsley, add the other ingredients and blend together well. The tahini gives this dressing a rounded, nutty flavor, and the cayenne and parsley add "zip."

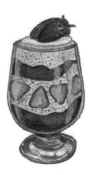

Dessert

Strawberry Rhubarb Chia Pudding
(Emily's Café, Pennington, NJ adapted from
food blog – The Year in Food – theyearinfood.com)
>   1/2 pound rinsed and diced rhubarb
>   1 pound rinsed and quartered strawberries
>   1/4 cup honey
>   1/4 cup water
>   1/2 vanilla bean
>   Juice of 1/2 lemon
>   1/4 cup chia seeds

1. In a medium pot, combine the strawberries, rhubarb, honey, and water. Slice the vanilla bean in half, scrape the seeds into the pot, and add the bean.

2. Bring to a boil, covered, then reduce heat to low, stirring occasionally. Simmer until the rhubarb has broken down, about 12 to 15 minutes. Blend with a hand held immersion blender or in a food processor. Set aside to cool.

3. When the compote is cooled to room temperature, add the chia seeds. Return to the fridge and allow to sit for at least two hours before eating.

Energy Balls (chef Madeleine Ezanno)
>   1 cup of cacao powder
>   2 cups of soaked almonds or pecans (for about 6-8 hrs)
>   1/2 cup coconut oil

2 tsp. of vanilla

pinch of salt

3/4 cup of coconut nectar

1/2 cup of maca or any super food

1. Blend ingredients in a food processor until it makes a dough
2. Roll into small balls and coat with chopped nuts (optional)

Recommended Reading, Watching, and Listening

Reading

Awareness

The Power of Now by Eckhart Tolle

The New Earth by Eckhart Tolle

Blink by Malcolm Gladwell

What is Light Body? by Archangel Ariel channeled by Tashira Tachi-ren

The Michael Handbook by Jose Stevens

Matrix Warrior – Being the One by Jake Horsley

A Beginners Guide to the Path of Ascension by Joshua David Stone

Power vs. Force by David R. Hawkins

Transcending the Levels of Consciousness by David R. Hawkins

I, Reality and Subjectivity by David R. Hawkins

Discovery of the Presence of GOD by David R. Hawkins

The Eye of the I by David R. Hawkins

Simplicity

Creating Sacred Space with Feng Shui by Karen Kingston

Choosing Simplicity by Linda Breen Pierce

Clutters Last Stand by Don Aslett
Your Money or Your Life by Joe Domniquez
Simplify Your Life by H. Norman Wright
Repacking Your Bags by David A. Shapiro
Simplify Your Life by Elaine St. James
Living the Simple Life by Elaine St. James
Inner Simplicity by Elaine St. James

Relating

Toxic People by Lillian Glass
Nasty People by Jay Carter
Pulling Your Own Strings by Wayne Dyer
Boundaries by Anne Katherine

Spiritual Philosophy

Walden or, Life in the Woods by Henry David Thoreau
Energy Blessings from the Stars by Irving Feurst
Infinite Self by Stuart Wilde
The Quickening by Stuart Wilde
The Force by Stuart Wilde
The Little Money Bible by Stuart Wilde
Whispering Winds of Change by Stuart Wilde
Weight Loss For the Mind by Stuart Wilde
The Ultimate Secret to Getting Absolutely Everything You Want by Mike
    Hernacki
Unlimited Power by Anthony Robbins
Awaken The Giant Within by Anthony Robbins
The Nature of Personal Reality by Jane Roberts

Nutrition/Detox

Skinny Bitch by Rory Freedman and Kim Barnouin
Spiritual Nutrition by Gabriel Cousens , M.D.

Rainbow Green Live Food Cuisine by Gabriel Cousens, M.D.
The Cure for All Disease by Hulda R. Clark
You are Not Sick You are Thirsty by F. Batmanghelidj
Colon Health Handbook by Robert Gray
Omnivore's Dilemma by Michael Pollan
In Defense of Food by Michael Pollan
Food Rules by Michael Pollan
Brain Maker by David Perlmutter, M.D.

Energy

Ancient Secret of The Fountain of Youth by Peter Kelder
Personal Power Through Awareness by Sanaya Roman Yoga Books
Light on Yoga by B.K.S.Iyengar
Light on Pranayama by B.K.S.Iyengar
The Yoga of Jesus by Paramahansa Yogananda
The Autobiography of Yogi by Paramahansa Yogananda
Awakening the Spine by Vanda Scaravelli

Watching
Food Documentaries

Food Matters
Forks Over Knives
Food Inc
Fresh
Fat, Sick and Nearly Dead
What The Health
Earthlings
GMO OMG
Food Choices
Kids Menu
The C Word
Hungry For Change
Sustainable

Awareness

Zeitgeist
Waking Life
What the Bleep Do You Know?

Listening

Your Wish is Your Command by Kevin Trudeau

Websites

The Non GMO Project's Free Shopping Guide
www.nonGMOProject.org
Check out the "Cooking Oil Comparison Chart" 02-22-12.pdf
https://eating rules.com/Cooking-Oil-Comparison-Chart
For the Dirty Dozen/Clean 15 list on your phone
www.EWG.org/FoodNews
Heavy Metals in Seafood
http://ewg.org/reserach/ewgsgood-seafood-guide
Institute for Responsible Non-GMO shopping guide for personal care
products, baby food, dairy, meat and more
www.nongmoshoppingguide.com/

Centers

Hippocrates Health Institute — http://hippocratesinst.org
Tree of Life — http://treeoflifecenterus.com
Gracious Living Oasis — http://www.gracevanberkum.com
Gerson Institute — https://gerson.org/gerpress/

Smartphone Applications

Buycott
Healthy Living
Fooducate
Waterlogged
ShopWell